Ketogenic Diet The Complete Cookbook

60+ Delicious Easy To Follow Meal Plan
Prep Recipes For Weight Loss, Prevent
Disease, Reset Your Metabolism, Boost
Brain Health, Living Long And Healthy!

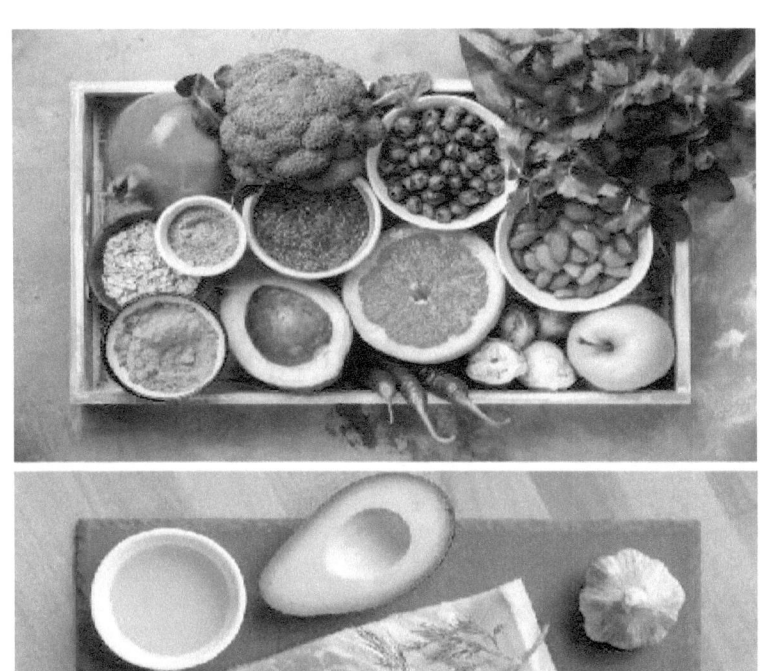

Table of Contents

Introduction

Ketogenic diets are diets in which a small number of carbohydrates (" low carb ") are consumed to very few carbohydrates ("no carb"). This means that the daily diet consists mainly of fish, meat, seafood, dairy products, nuts, kernels, legumes and low-sugar fruits and vegetables. However ,foods such as cereal products or potatoes are avoided.

The goal of a ketogenic diet is to put the body in a special metabolic state of " Ketosis " . This condition occurs when very few carbohydrates are added to the body (below 50g per day) and it has used up its glycogen stores (takes about 2 to 3 days).

The basis of a ketogenic diet - The macronutrients

In order to get an understanding of how ketogenic diet positively affect our body and our figure, we need to get an overview of the three macronutrients and their mode of action in the production of energy. We are talking about carbohydrates, fats and proteins.

✓ Proteins

Proteins are about 50% converted into combustible energy by our bodies. The remaining 50% are used for building new tissue, ie muscles, skin, hair. For this reason, high protein food sources play a tremendously important role as ketogenic foods. Proteins are important fuel in a low-carbohydrate phase and, on the other hand, they make the body beautifully taut, lean and attractive.

Proteins are literally considered a beauty nutrient. An amount of about 60-80 proteins per day (depending on the calorie requirement) gives the best results

✓ Fats

About 160-170 grams of fat should be consumed per day. In this way, you cover your calorie needs and give your body the necessary fuel.

Make sure, however, that the fatty acids are sourced from healthy sources like omega 3 fatty acids.

✓ Carbohydrates

Usually they are our main source of energy, which is why we usually cover about 50-60% of our daily requirement with carbohydrates. In our liver, they are converted into glucose, which is then available as a fast source of energy.

On the other hand, carbohydrates are the fattening thing, because our main foods such as rice, pasta and potatoes consist of up to 70% carbohydrates. This entices us to consume more energy than we really need, and as soon as that happens, the body converts the carbohydrates into fat deposits (stored energy).

✓ The difficulty in losing weight with carbohydrates:

The body burns in the calorie deficit, first the remaining glucose stores and only then the fat reserves. As a result, you'll need longer for the weight loss process and have to budget for an increased calorie deficit. Both are not much fun.

You can not consume more than 50 grams of carbs per day. To follow the keto diet properly , you should maintain 30 grams per day(optimal value)

Ketogenic diet - The principle

The weight loss effect comes about as follows:

As soon as the body has less than 50 grams of carbohydrates a day,it is forced to pull the energy from other sources . For this purpose, the liver produces so-called ketone bodies from the consumed fatty acids, which alternatively act as a fast source of energy.

In this state of "ketosis" is actively and almost exclusively fat used as an energy source, whereby the body's fat reserves are targeted tapped as soon as the body is in a calorie deficit (what else is the body not left, because there is no other source of energy more). The ketogenic diet is literally a fat burner.

Very important: Also for the ketogenic diet, you must absolutely adhere to a calorie deficit. The hip gold and belly fat can only be tapped if the body has received fewer calories through the diet at the end of the day than it actually needs.

Water loss at the beginning of the Ketogenic diet

The main reason for the relatively high weight loss at the beginning of ketogenic diets are the emptying glycogen stores of the body. All carbohydrates are first broken down by the body into glucose (glucose) and then either consumed or stored as glycogen in muscles and liver.

This glycogen in the body, which brings it to a total of 200-400 g, binds again 600-1200 g of water. If the reservoirs empty, the bound water is also eliminated . It comes to a corresponding weight loss. If you eat carbohydrates again, the glycogen stores fill up again and water is bound again. The weight goes up.

✓ The calorie deficit decides

If carbohydrates are missing as an energy supplier, the body burns more fat and amino acids , but these may just as well come from the food as from its cells .

If the energy balance is balanced or positive, meaning that eating enough fat or protein to absorb enough or excessive calories, the body does not need to tap the fat cells to sustain its operation - ketosis or not. How much fat is burned in ketogenic diets, therefore, mainly determines the calorie deficit .

Which foods are allowed?

As with any diet, the list of foods that are banned is quite long. But what foods are allowed when choosing this particular diet? Mostly it's about food that contains protein and fats.

- Meat (steak, bacon, turkey, chicken, ham, red meat)

- Fish (trout, tuna, salmon, mackerel)

- Nuts (walnuts, almonds)

- eggs

- Seeds (pumpkin seeds, chia seeds, flax seeds)

- Dairy products (cream, cheese, butter)

- Spices (pepper, salt, herbs)

- Vegetables (green vegetables, onions, tomatoes, avocado)

- Healthy oils (coconut oil, virgin olive oil, avocado oil)

Which foods are banned?

The diet also has a long list of what you should not eat. Especially sugars and foods high in carbohydrates are prohibited. Do not eat:

- Starchy: rice, bread, lentils, pasta, potatoes

- Cereals: All Whole Grains , Spelled, Wheat, Oats, Couscous, Oatmeal, and Bulgur

- Soy and soy products

- Sweet: everything that contains sugar

- Alcohol: Beer, Cocktails, Cyder

- Highly processed food: This usually contains a lot of glucose and saturated fat

Who needs a ketogenic diet?

In conventional medicine, the ketogenic diet is used very successfully for the treatment of epilepsy (especially in children) that do not respond to medication. Some clinics offer the ketogenic diet as an adjunctive nutrition therapy for cancer patients. Behind this is the idea that the metabolism in cancer is often changed, and the body needs a lot more fat and protein than without the disease. Cancer patients very often also suffer from an inflammatory reaction that promotes cancer growth. Ketone bodies have an anti-inflammatory effect. Carbohydrates promote inflammation and serve as an energy source, especially the cancer cells - they need them to grow quickly. In this respect, a ketogenic diet strengthens the patient without feeding the cancer growth while reducing the cancer-promoting inflammatory reactions.

Recently, there is evidence that ketosis can halt the progression of Alzheimer's and partially reverse existing limitations. Positive effects were also observed in the nerve disease multiple sclerosis (MS) . In all these applications: The ketogenic diet must be calculated individually according to one's own preferences and monitored by professionals.

✓ Ketogenic diet against overweight

As the dietary change towards ketosis boosts and improves fat burning, the ketogenic diet is also used against high obesity . The "trick" of the body to activate fat as an energy source in carbohydrate deficiency . If you want to follow a ketogenic diet, you should definitely get the necessary know-how from professionals - for example in specialized health clinics and rehabilitation facilities, where ketogenic cooking can be learned under the supervision of a doctor and expert diet instructions in the in-house teaching kitchen.

Quick Slimming Tips –Ketosis

Ketosis is a metabolic condition in which the body degrades body fat due to insulin deficiency and uses it for energy. Ketosis is also called "starvation metabolism" because this effect also occurs when not enough food is absorbed and the body is forced to use up its fat stores.

However, a permanent fasting seems not desirable. Although short-term fasting has many health benefits, but if you want to lose a lot of weight, it is not advisable and it is also difficult to keep going for months without eating anything.

After all, the body needs to be supplied with a variety of vitamins and minerals to stay healthy and efficient. Therefore, the ketogenic diet imitates a kind of fasting condition for the body.

The negative consequences of the keto diet

✓ Not much carbohydrates and lots of fat

That's the motto of the keto diet. The effects of this diet on the body are not always positive. From the "keto flu" to libido loss .

It almost seems as if everyone is currently a fan of the keto diet. You can always read something about the positive effects and easy implementation of the diet. But before you decide to try Keto for yourself, you should also get to know the negative "side effects".

✓ loss of libido

The ketogenic diet is based on an extremely low carbohydrate, high-fat diet. This is to bring the metabolism in a specific state - the ketosis - which makes the body more efficient in burning fat.

Ketosis has positive effects on weight loss, but not in other areas: recently, keto has been increasingly criticized because some experts say that the diet can cause changes in the libido.

✓ The keto flu

Many have already heard of keto flu, which often occurs at the beginning of the diet. It can manifest itself in several ways: headache , weakness, irritability, constipation, nausea and vomiting are common symptoms.

Once the body is in a state of ketosis after some time - burning fat instead of glucose - the keto diet works and the withdrawal symptoms go back. But you probably feel pretty bad at first. The reason: The body must first get used to the lower carbohydrate intake.

With the onset of the keto diet, the body is switching from using sugar as an energy source to using the stored fat in the body," explains Rahnama. "When fat is broken down, the body produces ketones, which are then removed by the body through frequent and increased urination .This can lead to dehydration and flu-like symptoms.

✓ yoyo effect

The keto diet leads more often than other diets to the yo-yo effect , because people have difficulty adhering to the restrictive dietary rules. There are only a few long-term studies on the ketogenic diet, possibly because the diet is so difficult to follow that people can not stick to it over a long period of time.

Other effects of the yo-yo effect, according to experts may be bad breath, fatigue, constipation, irregular menstrual cycles, decreased bone density, and sleep problems.

Is keto suitable for me?

Keto is not particularly recommendable for certain groups of people: it should be advised against hypertension, diabetes or other chronic diseases.This diet could change so much for the metabolic and other body systems that it would even change the effectiveness of a medication.

You should consult a doctor before starting the keto diet and have him monitor the diet change. Perhaps the electrolyte balance should be supported by supplements that a physician can prescribe.

Tips for Exercising When on a Ketogenic Diet

A lot of things happen when you are exercising. Some of these are good for your health and others are not so good - like when you exercise excessively.

Exercise is a stressor. While it can be a good stressor, it can however cause your adrenals to go into overdrive. This situation increases your insulin levels and therefore reduces your ability to lose weight .

When exercising, your insulin levels goes up while your hunger reduces. However, this often results in a significant reduction in blood sugar levels which results to you becoming hungrier .

It is important to note that even a moderate increase in insulin levels causes a significant lowering of fat loss or lipolysis .

One problem we have when we want to lose weight is that we focus so much on the numbers showing on the scale. We almost unconsciously forget about the most important thing which is losing body fat .

We have more than 80 percent of our body fat stored in fat cells. To be able to get rid of these stored fat, one would need to burn it for energy production .

However, before your body can start burning your stored fats for energy, your need to be in a negative fat balance. This is condition in which you are burning more fat off than you are actually taking in through your diet.

If your body has become used to burning fat for energy , it can now use both body fat and dietary fat for energy . This is one of the key powers of using a ketogenic diet for losing weight.

If you do not increase your dietary fat intake but increase the amount of energy your body needs through increasing your exercise intensity, your body will get almost all of that energy from burning body fat.

However , if your body is fueled with carbs , you will mostly be burning glucose for energy. This makes it a lot difficult for your body to burn and lose body fat.

It is however important to understand that while exercise can help you lose weight , it is more important to get the diet right first .

When you get the diet right, such a by using a well-designed ketogenic diet, your body will start tapping into its fat deposits for generating its energy. This is what effectively enables you to start burning and losing body fat .

Once your body gets used to the ketogenic diet, you will start feeling more energetic. At such a point, you will be better positioned to adjust your menus in order to start building strength and muscles .

When you get to this point during the "standard ketogenic" diet, you can then alter the diet to either a "targeted" or a "cyclical" ketogenic diet . These versions of the ketogenic diet allow more carbohydrate consumption to enable you engage in more exercises for longer .

    ✓ Targeted Ketogenic Diet

The Targeted Ketogenic Diet allows you to ingest more carbs around your exercise period. This form of the diet allows you to engage in high-intensity exercise while still remaining in ketosis .

The carb intake within this window provides your muscles with the necessary glucose to effectively engage in your workouts . The extra glucose should normally be used up during this window of about 30 minutes and should not affect your overall metabolism.

The Targeted Ketogenic Diet is designed for beginners or intermittent exercisers. The TKD allows a slight increase in your carb consumption. However, it does not kick you out ketosis and causes no shock to your system.

    ✓ Cyclical Ketogenic Diet

The Cyclical Ketogenic Diet is more appropriate for advanced athletes and bodybuilders. It is generally used for maximum muscle building results .

There is however a strong tendency for other individuals to end up adding some body fat. This is because it is easy to overeat while using the Cyclical Ketogenic Diet (CKD).

In this version of the ketogenic diet, the individual follows the standard ketogenic diet for 5 or 6 days. He or she is then allowed to eat increased amounts of carbohydrate for 1 or 2 days .

As a caution, it can take a beginner close to 3 weeks to fully get back into ketosis if he or she attempts the CKD . It requires real commitment and advanced exercise levels to successfully carry out a CKD .

The aim of the Cyclical Ketogenic Diet is to temporarily switch out of ketosis. This window gives the body the opportunity to refill the amount of glycogen in the muscles to enable it undertake the next cycle of intense workouts.

Therefore, there must be a complete depletion of the resultant glycogen build up during the subsequent workouts in order to get back into ketosis. The intensity of your planned workout will consequently determine the amount of increased carbohydrate intake.

✓ Cardio Exercises

When you exercise at an intense rate, a lot of amazing things happen to your body.

When you engage in cardiovascular exercises , they help to improve the efficiency of your heart and lungs. This also helps to increase the rate at which your body burns energy and over time this will lead to weight loss.

Engaging in cardio exercise causes many metabolic changes that positively affect fat metabolism.

Cardiovascular exercises helps to increase oxygen delivery through improved blood flow. This way, body cells are able to more effectively oxidize and burn fat.

This also has the effect of increasing the number of oxidative enzymes. Consequently, the speed at which fatty acids are transported to the mitochondria to be burned for energy is greatly increased .

During cardio exercises, the sensitivity of muscles and fat cells to epinephrine is greatly increased. This increases the amount of triglycerides that are released into the blood and muscles to be burned for energy.

✓ Strength Training

Strength training helps to improve your moods while also helping to build healthy bones. It also helps you to develop an overall strong and healthy body.

Using a well-designed ketogenic will help you preserve your muscles even when carrying our strength training . Muscles are built with protein and not fat or carbs. Also, given the fact that protein oxidation is less in a ketogenic diet, engaging in strength training should not be a problem .

You need to challenge your body with heavy weights to really see results and get a stronger body.

✓ Interval Training

Interval training is simply alternating intervals of high-intensity and low-intensity workouts. It is simply for you to : go fast, go slow, and repeat.

While sounding so simple, interval training is one the most powerful ways to burn body fat quickly. Apart from burning fat while carrying out interval training, the "afterburn effect" stimulates your metabolism for a longer period of time.

✓ Circuit Training: Cardio + Strength

Circuit training is basically the combining of cardiovascular exercises with strength training exercises. This combination helps to provide all-over fitness benefits.

This form of exercising combines cardio exercises such a jogging and a resistance workout without allowing a resting period between them. The lack of rest in-between both exercises make circuit training as effective as a cardio-based high-intensity interval training workout .

✓ Yoga

The exercise benefits of yoga really come from its ability to help the body reduce levels of stress hormones and also increase insulin sensitivity .

Yoga helps you to consciously connect with your body. This connection can translate into you being more mindful of how your body works and changing even your eating habits .

The Benefits of Mixing MCT Oil Into Your Ketogenic Diet Plan

In life, we're always talking about must haves. If you're driving a high end car, you must have the top of the line motor oil coursing through its cylinders. If you're competing at a high level in a track competition, state of the art running shoes are a must have. When you're celebrating a huge *q*uarter at the office, the finest bourbon is a must have. I would submit to you, that if you're serious about a ketogenic lifestyle , MCT Oil is a must have.

MCT Oil provides a heavy dose of the very fuels that turn your body into - and keep it - a fat burning machine. Unlike LCTs, MCTs bypass much of the digestion process that others fats go through. MCTs act in an almost carb-like manner in how they're sent directly to the liver , where they are used for energy.

There are many reasons why MCT makes perfect sense for your Ketogenic Diet, but help you understand how they can play an essential role in your nutrition, we've some of the main benefits of MCT Oil in your Ketogenic Diet plan.

✓ MCT OIL HELPS YOUR GET INTO KETOSIS FASTER

As you already know, MCTs go to your liver, and act in a "carb-like" manner that LCTs do not have the ability to do . This means that you can theoretically kickstart Ketosis by following these steps :

1. Fast with no breakFAST.

If you've been out of Ketosis for awhile and you want to efficiently get back into a fat burning state, a mix of fasting and MCT Oil will do the job. Just eat a very low carb dinner, or even skip dinner , and then wake up and don't eat breakfast! Instead, drink a cup of coffee , and put a tablespoon or two of MCT Oil into your coffee and head out!

The shot of MCT, plus the already fasted state of your body will have you back into Ketosis quicker than if you tried to just slowly eat your way back into Ketosis (i.e. nutritional Ketosis). It's also worth adding that the energy you get from the MCT Oil and the coffee will be unlike what you were used to : the MCTs provide a prolonged energy that isn't comparable to energy derived from glycogen.

2. Meal replacement with MCT Oil

Another benefit that comes from using MCT Oil in your Ketogenic Diet plan is using it as a meal replacement.

This somewhat resembles the previous point of fasting with MCT Oil, but the difference is that you're still eating other regular Ketogenic meals, except your replacing (at least) one of those meals with some MCT Oil.

One of the benefits of MCT Oil is its ability to satiate your appetite. So while it sounds initially scary to just depend a few tablespoons of oil for a meal replacement, your body will become accustomed as you do it more and more. The MCTs will act as replacement for what's normally there (glycogen) and your fierce-badger-hunger cravings will lessen .

In our fast paced, 21st century lifestyle, the benefits of being able to remain in Ketosis while only slurping a few tablespoons of MCTs cannot be overstated.

3. Ramp up your Ketogenic dishes with MCT

MCT Oil's versatility is amazing. Let's say you're already in Ketosis, but you're about to eat a salad for your daily carbs, and you want to keep it 100 on the Keto life. It's easy! Just use MCT for a base to your dressing, and you can rest assured that you'll still be burning fat after you've downed your greens !

Another way to use MCTs in your favorite Ketogenic meals is to use it as a replacement for regular oil in baking! There's a whole ocean of Keto baking recipes out there, so why not double down and use MCT instead of regular coconut oil?!

But what if you're not baking? What if you're out for a jog and you want to implement the energy efficiency of MCT Oil? How about a nice Keto "sports drink"?! All you have to do is it to water , and then squeeze in some lemon juice, and you'll have a healthier, non-sugary sports drink for long workouts in the sun!

There are many ways to skin a cat , and there's also many ways to amplify your Ketogenic Diet. MCTs are essential to your body transforming into a fat burning machine. Unfortunately , you're not always going to be able to get the proper amounts from a diet alone - you'll need a boost, and MCT Oil is that boost.

Life is full of "must haves," and your diet does not fall out of the realm of this mantra. If you want to live a truly Ketogenic lifestyle, you're going to have invest in the right fuels, and implement them in the most efficient ways possible. So what's the benefit of MCT to your Ketogenic Diet plan? The answer: efficiency. An efficient diet, which feeds an efficient lifestyle, that ultimately gives you more time to do the things you love.

The best fast slimming Tips for the Success in Ketosis.

√ KEEP AN EYE ON CALORIE INTAKE

To lose weight, you should be aware of how many calories you should eat to lose fat. You will only lose weight if you make a calorie deficit, so eat less than you consume.

√ DISTRIBUTE MACRONUTRIENTS CORRECTLY

In the ketogenic diet, however, not only is the number of calories crucial, but also the macronutrient distribution of carbohydrates, fats and proteins. Maximum 20g of carbs per day and 15-25% protein and the rest fat, about 70-80%.

If you practice sports, you are welcome to consume 25% protein. However, it should be ensured that the protein is distributed evenly over all meals, as one too many at a time can stimulate insulin secretion. This would break the ketosis.

If you consume a keto diet, but still hungry all the time, it may be a sign of too much protein. Remember, the ketogenic diet requires very little carbohydrate, lots of fat and moderate protein intake.

✓ SPORTS

If you pay attention to the first two points and want to get a little bit more out of your diet, you will not get around sport. Movement should generally be part of everyday life .

Of course, you do not have to go to the gym for hours every day, but 20-30 minutes 3 times a week should be completed.

The important thing is that it makes you fun. However, I recommend you more strength sports. The more muscle you have, the higher your basal metabolic rate, even if you're not doing any sports. So you burn more calories in the future. Even when doing nothing.

✓ INTERMITTENT FASTING - FOR MAXIMUM FAT BURNING

If you've already implemented the above tips and doing regular exercise, there's another option that will boost fat loss fast. You do not have to eat less or do more sport, instead you only change the times to eat.

This method is called intermittent fasting. For starters, we recommend a 9-hour meal window and a 15-hour fasting phase. When exactly you eat is up to you, but many people find it easier to skip breakfast.

FOR EXAMPLE;

Get up at 7 o'clock, first meal at 11 o'clock and the last one at 20 o'clock. The fasting phase takes place mainly at night and is quite easy to hold on. Depending on how you can easily integrate them into your daily routine, you can also shift the time you eat.

In the morning until the first meal you should drink a lot of water, unsweetened tea or black coffee. In the fasting phase, however, no calories are recorded.

✓ HOWEVER, THIS TYPE OF DIET IS NOT SUITABLE FOR EVERYONE:

People with a lot of stress and pregnant women should refrain from doing so. In general, it may be difficult for women intermittently to fast, the prolonged deprivation of food may cause an imbalance of hormones, as the body interprets fasting as stress.

What are the risks of the ketogenic diet?

From a medical point of view, the following are the risks and side effects of ketogenic diet:

✓ Increase in cholesterol level

✓ kidney damage

✓ Increased risk of cancer (breast and large intestine)

✓ bone damage

✓ heart disease

✓ arteriosclerosis

✓ constipation

✓ halitosis

✓ nausea

✓ yoyo effect

Ketogenic diet and weight loss

losing weight is quite easy with the ketogenic diet . Sugar, carbohydrates and alcohol are absolutely eliminated . Energy is gained from fat. In ketosis, the body's own fat reserves are attacked to maintain performance. This has the effect of being able to lose up to three kilos in one week. Of course, this varies depending on the starting position.

Some studies even suggest that the high-fat diet is more effective than a low-fat diet. For example, one study shows that subjects who ate ketogenically lost twice as much body fat and weight than the peer group. This had calorie-reduced and low-fat diet.

However, it should also be noted that a too rapid weight reduction can lead to the yo-yo effect . Therefore, you should be aware of the food choices. You can also make the daily intake of high-fat foods healthy. Because a high-fat diet does not automatically mean masses of sausage and meat in it. Healthy nutrition is also very important here.

Ketogenic nutritional plan for one day

The ketogenic diet is unfamiliar to most at first . But there are many delicious recipes that make the diet easy. In addition, they can support a healthy metabolism. To be able to supply both body and brain sufficiently, the diet for one day could look like this:

√ Breakfast:

All breads are not allowed, so you have to find alternatives. Scrambled eggs with bacon are cooked very quickly. In addition, this food is a real power-start for the day.

√ Lunch:

Salad as a side dish is always. You could eat a hearty steak for that.

Evening: To avoid going to bed with too heavy a stomach, fish is a good solution. Salmon provides valuable fatty acids and can be combined well with vegetables - such as spinach.

√ Snacks:

Make sure not to overpower. If you still feel like having a snack, nuts are ideal. For the ketogenic diet are especially hazelnuts, walnuts and almonds.

FAQ's

✓ How do you get into ketosis - When do ketone bodies form?

Ketone bodies are formed when fatty acids are burned or metabolized in the absence of glucose (glucose). If it has ketone bodies in the blood you have too little glucose available to completely burn fats. If you reduce the carbohydrates in the diet very much, you will get into ketosis.

✓ When do you "fly out of ketosis"?

Quite simply, if your metabolism has enough glucose to completely burn the needed fats. If you consume enough carbohydrates for your individual needs, your metabolism will stop producing ketone bodies. That does not mean that you will not lose weight anymore. It does not mean that no more fat burning takes place. It only means that no ketone bodies are produced anymore.

✓ When is ketosis dangerous?

As long as you have not more than 5 mmol / L ketone body in the blood, the whole thing is unproblematic. Your body will not produce more than 5 mmol / L even if you are healthy.

This is different for example in type 1 diabetics and in certain types of type 2 diabetics. There, significantly higher ketone body levels can occur, which can then be life-threatening in the context of so-called ketoacidosis (hyperacidity with ketone bodies)

Ketosis and Ketoacidosis

For many, ketosis may have many benefits - for some, the formation of ketone bodies can be dangerous in certain metabolic situations.

Ketosis must be clearly distinguished from the term keto acidosis. The blood plasma concentration of the ketone bodies in a ketosis is between 0.5 and 5 mmol / L and affects the pH of the blood in a physiological context. In a ketoacidosis, however, creates a dangerous acidity of the blood.

Fat is increasingly broken down and there are many free fatty acids in the blood. This also increases the concentration of acetyl-CoA from which ketone bodies are made. This can cause acidosis. Acidosis is a lowering of the pH. Two of the three above-mentioned ketone bodies dissociate, ie they separate and the pH drops. You can read more about the pH of the body in the acid-base balance article .

In contrast, ketoacidosis occurs mainly in patients with diabetes mellitus type 1 and is caused by an imbalance of certain hormones (insulin, glucagon or cortisol). The complication is the result of a severe insulin deficiency , to which the body reacts with the release of stress hormones (eg cortisol), which increases the release of glucose into the bloodstream. The body increasingly forms ketone body, which leads to acidification of the body. As a result, it can lead to the body drying out and derailment of the electrolyte budget.

Conspicuous with ketoacidotic patients is the acetone smell (smells like rotten apples) in the air. An untreated ketoacidosis leads to a coma and thus the death of the patient! With acetone odor and a high blood sugar level, a patient immediately belongs to the nearest hospital.

8 Delicious Fruits That You Can Eat With A Ketogenic Diet

You try the keto diet to lose weight, but all that butter, cheese and meat can be heavy at times. And so lighten your meals with some fruit seems like a wise choice, is not it?

Not so fast! With this high-fat diet, carbohydrates should not exceed 5% of your caloric intake to stay in ketosis (that is, a state where your body burns fat to make energy rather than carbohydrates). And (big scoop attention) the fruits are quite rich in carbohydrates. But following a diet low in carbohydrates and high in fat like the ketogenic diet does not mean you have to give up all the fruits and vegetables.

Take the example of blueberries: a 150g container contains about 17.4g of net carbohydrate (ie total carbohydrate minus fiber), which is about the equivalent of a carbohydrate. whole day of carbohydrates with the keto diet (we are supposed to eat less than 20 g net carbs a day). So, in principle, you can not eat most fruits with a keto diet. In addition, the sweetest fruits are usually the tastiest ones like peaches and melons. But there is not necessarily need to get rid of all the fruits in the keto diet. Here are some fruits that can be consumed in moderation without breaking your ketosis.

1.Avocado

Most people "think" that avocados and tomatoes are vegetables,but technically they are both fruits.And as they are fruits, and very delicious, we included them in our list of low carbohydrate fruits. Avocados contain 8.5 grams of carbohydrate per 100 grams,which is a bit high. But the good news is that they have 6.7 grams of dietary fiber (oh yeah), which reduces the amount of net carbs to 1.8 g.If you have a ketogenic diet with little carbohydrate ... there is really little food that can be compared to the avocado. They have an excellent taste and are filled with good fats.

There are endless ways to prepare and eat avocados. We can eat them on our salads, all alone for lunch, on a hamburger without bread or guacamole. Honestly, we can not find a better food?

2. Tomato

Another fruit (at least scientifically) that is often mistaken for a vegetable. Raw tomatoes contain 3.89 grams of carbohydrate per 100 grams. They also contain (on average) 1.2 grams of dietary fiber, giving a total of 2.69 grams of net carbohydrate. Tomatoes can be eaten raw in salad, keto chili, with a avocado in a hamburger without bread, and so on.There are really tons of different ways to add tomatoes to your diet.

A little warning. Tomatoes can cause inflammation (and therefore an increase in blood sugar) in those who suffer from autoimmune diseases. Indeed, tomatoes are part of the family nightshade and for some people, they can cause significant allergic reactions.

These delicious fruits should be avoided if you follow an Auto-Immune Protocol (AIP).

3. Blackberry

This may surprise you, but blackberries are one of the lowest carbohydrate fruits (or berries). These small berries contain a total of 9.61 grams of carbohydrate per 100 grams,which is a bit high.Luckily, they also contain a lot of dietary fiber: 5.3 grams. This brings the total net carbs to 4.31 grams, which remains reasonable. In season, add some wild blackberries (if possible) to your favorite salads or as a snack in summer.

4. Raspberry

Raspberries are also part of the family of berries that do not have a lot of carbohydrates. They contain 11.94 grams of carbohydrates per 100 grams. The good surprise is that they contain 6.5 grams of dietary fiber, which makes us a total net carb of 5.44 grams.

Raspberries are perfect as a snack, on a salad, in a smoothie or on keto pancakes,there is only the embarrassment of choice! They are also great because they can easily be frozen in season and used later when they are no longer readily available.

5. Strawberry

There are not many more pleasant things in life than fresh strawberries on a hot summer day. The big news is that you can continue to eat these delicious berries with a low carbohydrate diet like the keto diet. These bright red berries contain 7.68 grams of carbohydrate per 100 grams, including 2.0 grams of dietary fiber, bringing the total net carbs to 5.68 grams.

 Just like blackberries and raspberries, strawberries are excellent on salads, for dessert, in smoothies, as a snack.

6. Olives

Wait, what? Olives are fruits? Well yes, these are fruits that can also be enjoyed with a keto diet. 10 small olives contain only 1.5 grams of carbohydrates. The fat content is 3 grams per 10 olives and on top of that, it is an excellent source of sodium, which is very important when following a low carbohydrate diet. Rich in antioxidants (polyphenols), these stars of the Mediterranean diet are excellent for keeping the body healthy. Do not deprive yourself then as an aperitif!

7. Lemon

This fruit (citrus) alkaline is perfectly compatible with a keto diet. Lemons are low in carbohydrates and are an excellent source of vitamin C, potassium and calcium. On top of that, they will give your taste buds a little pleasure and can do wonders for your weight loss goals. Indeed, citric acid has detoxifying and diuretic effects that have always been recognized.

With less than half a gram of sugar per quarter of lemon, do not hesitate to add it in your infusions or your water. You can also add lemon juice to your sauce or some zest for meat or fish roasts.

8. Coconut

Coconut is one of the most generous sources of good fats and is also very low in carbohydrates. 50 g of grated coconut contains only 3.7 g of carbohydrates. Therefore, they can be included in your keto diet in moderation.And of course, you can also consume (it is even recommended!) Coconut oil, coconut vinegar and coconut flour for your keto pastries.

KETOGENIC RECIPES

Keto Breakfast Recipes

- **Keto Egg Muffins With Sausage And Veggies**

These Keto egg muffins are packed with protein and veggie,they are so easy to make and grab on the go and include everything in one neat little package.

Ingredients:

- 8 oz Pork Breakfast Sausage
- 1 Tbsp Extra Virgin Olive Oil
- ½ Sweet Onion (thinly sliced)
- ¾ Cup Red Bell Peppers (chopped or thinly sliced, any color)
- 1 1/2 Cups Fresh Spinach (packed)
- 1 tsp Fresh Oregano (chopped or ½ t. dry oregano)
- 9 Eggs
- Ground Pepper
- ¾ tsp Real Salt
- ¼ Cup Milk

Instructions:

1. Preheat oven to 350 F degrees. Grease a 12 cup, regular size muffin pan.

2. Place the ground sausage in a sauté pan and heat on medium high. Break up the pork into crumbles with a spatula as it cooks.

3. When the pork is half way cooked, add 1 T. of olive oil, onions, peppers, and oregano to the pan. Saute until the onion is translucent. Add the spinach to the pan and cover with a lid. Cook for 30 seconds, remove the lid and toss the ingredients. Spinach should be wilted but still bright green. Remove from heat.

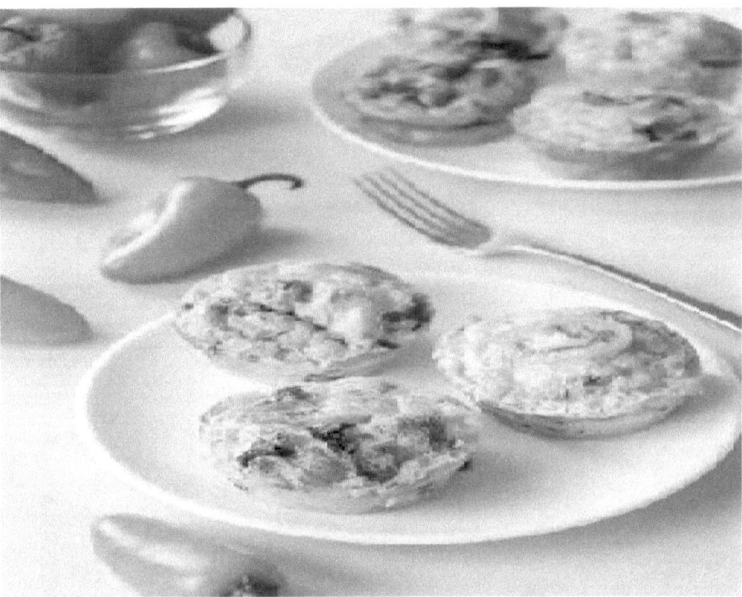

4. Place the eggs in a large mixing bowl along with the pepper, salt, and milk. Whisk together until eggs are well beaten.

5. Add the sausage and vegetables to the egg mixture and mix in until well distributed.

6. Divide the mixture between the greased muffin tins (12 total), making sure that each tin has a somewhat equal ratio of eggs/fillings.

7. Bake in preheated oven for 18-20 minutes. Cool for a few minutes and remove from tins, loosening the edges first with a knife.

* **Low-Carb Crustless Breakfast Tarts**

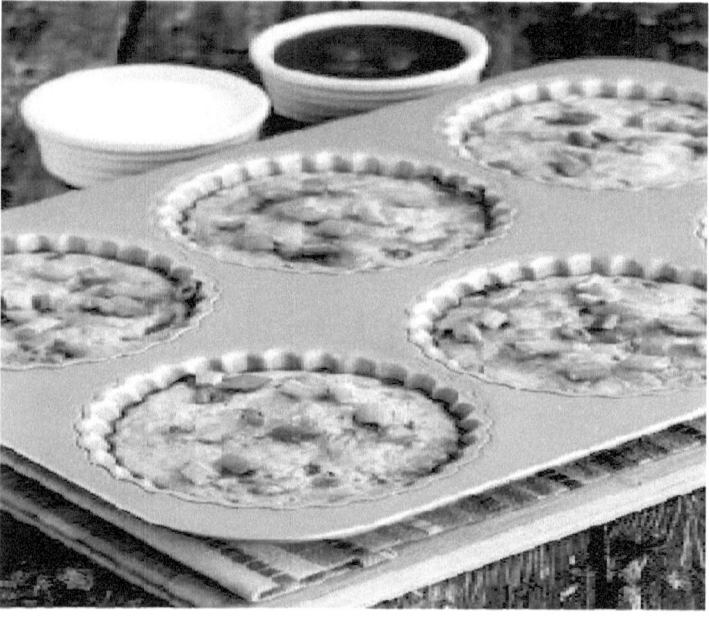

Ingredients:

- 1 large red bell pepper, seeds and stem removed and cut into short strips (If you prefer, replace the red bell pepper with a 12 oz. jar of roasted red peppers, or a mix of red and yellow peppers. Drain the jarred peppers well; no need to saute them.)

- 1 – 2 tsp. olive oil (depending on your pan)

- 1 can (4 oz.) diced green chiles (This wasn't much spice, but you can use less than a full can if you're making for kids or don't want them spicy.)

- 2 green onions, thinly sliced

- 1/4 cup sour cream, whisked to soften

- 1/4 tsp. ground cumin

- 1 tsp. Spike Seasoning (Or use any all-purpose seasoning that's good with eggs if you don't have Spike.)

- fresh-ground black pepper to taste

- 6 eggs

- 1/2 – 3/4 cup grated Mexican Blend cheese

- additional sour cream or salsa or thinly sliced green onions for serving, optional

Instructions:

1. Preheat oven to 375F/190C. Spray the tart pan (or large muffin cups) with non-stick spray or olive oil.

2. Cut out the stem and seeds from the red bell pepper and cut it into short strips.

3. Heat the olive oil in a non-stick pan over medium-high heat, add the red peppers, and cook 2-3 minutes, just until they barely start to soften. Then add the can of diced green chiles and cook about 2 minutes more.

4. Slice green onions while peppers and chiles are cooking.

5. Divide the pepper mixture among the tart wells and add a generous pinch of green onion to each one, topped with a generous pinch of grated cheese.

6. (If you prefer to use red peppers from a jar, dump the jar of roasted peppers into a colander placed in the sink and let the peppers drain well while you slice the green onions. When the peppers are drained, blot dry with paper towels, remove any seeds or membranes, and slice peppers into short strips. Divide the pepper strips, green chiles if using, and sliced green onions among the tart wells and top with a generous pinch of grated cheese.)

7. Put the sour cream in a large glass measuring cup (or a bowl with a pour spout) and whisk the sour cream with a fork. Add the ground cumin, Spike Seasoning, and fresh-ground black pepper and stir to combine.

8. Then add the eggs two at a time, whisking with the fork between each pair of eggs to combine the yolks and whites and mix the eggs with the sour cream. (Don't worry if the eggs and sour cream are not perfectly combined.)

9. Divide the egg mixture evenly among the tarts, pouring it over the peppers/cheese. Use a fork to gently stir each one so the cheese, peppers, and green onions are well-distributed in the eggs.

10. Bake tarts 25-27 minutes, or until the eggs are completely set and the top is starting to get lightly browned. (If you're using a muffin pan where the wells are less than 4 inches in diameter, you might have to increase the cooking time a little.)

11. Serve hot, with a dollop of sour cream and some salsa on top if desired.

12. These crustless breakfast tarts will keep at least a week in the refrigerator and can be microwaved or reheated in a toaster oven. (Don't microwave too long or the eggs will get rubbery.)

- **Mini Egg Quiches**

Ingredients:

- 1.75 eggs
- 0.38 plum tomatoes
- 1/12 cups mozzarella cheese
- 1/24 cups pepper jack
- 1/24 cups sweet vidalia onion
- 1/24 cups sliced pickled jalapenos
- 1/12 cups soppressata salami
- 1/24 cups heavy cream

- 0.13 tbsps olive oil

- 0.13 tsps salt

- 0.13 tsps pepper

- 1/16 tsps cayenne

Instructions:

1. Preheat your oven to 325°F and grease a 15" x 11" muffin tin.

2. Chop up and combine all your ingredients in a mixing bowl and season them with the salt, pepper and cayenne. Got a favorite spice? Add it into the mix! These things are bursting with different flavors. The more the merrier. Extra tip: if you like some crunch, try frying up the salami first and then throw it into your egg mixture.

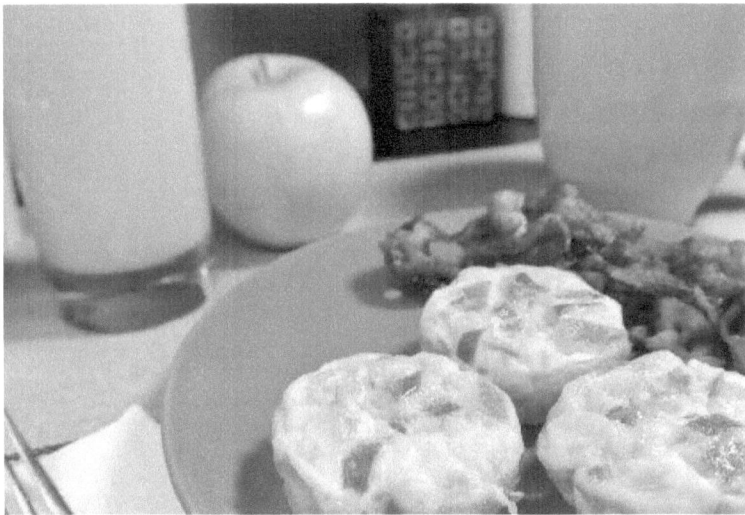

3. Crack all the eggs into the bowl and whisk them up until everything is well combined

4. Add in your heavy cream and whisk once again. Along with the cheese, the heavy cream will give your eggs fluffiness and moisture. Not to mention, heavy cream is very keto friendly.

5. You're ready to pour! The ensure all the mini quiches are roughly the same size, use an ice cream scooper to measure and ladle. Make sure to leave some room for the quiches to rise. Keep in mind, the bigger the scoops, the more they'll rise.

6. Stick your batch in the oven (middle rack) for about 25 minutes or until you see your desired golden brown color appear.

7. You should have no problem popping them out as they probably shrunk away from their tins a bit.

8. Your mini quiches are ready to eat! Serve hot with bacon, toast, fruit or your favorite omelette pairing.

- **Scrambled eggs**

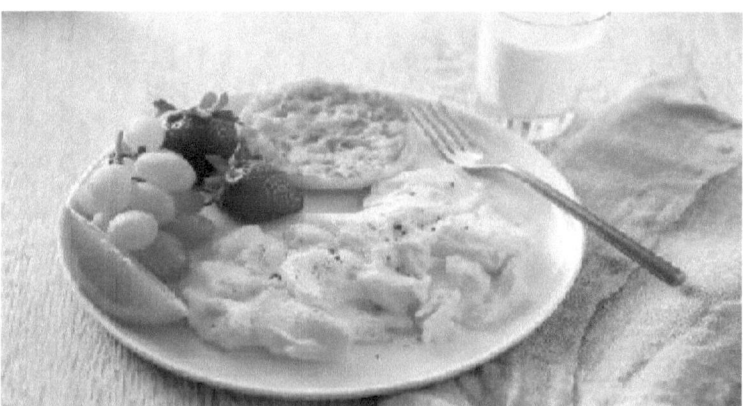

Ingredients :

- 2 eggs

- 30 g butter

- Salt and ground black peppe

Instructions

- Beat the eggs together with some salt and pepper using a fork.

- Melt the butter in a nonstick skillet over medium heat. Look closely: butter does not turn golden!

- Pour the eggs into the pan and mix for 1-2 minutes until they are creamy and cooked a little less than you like. Remember that the eggs will continue to cook even once you put them on your plate.

Tips!

These creamy eggs pair well with many popular low carb dishes. Of course, there is the option of eating them with classic accompaniments such as bacon or sausage, but there are other great options such as salmon, avocado, cold cuts and cheese (cheddar, fresh mozzarella or feta).

- **Keto eggs with avocado and bacon**

Sail to a ketogenic breakfast with this fancy touch with eggs and bacon. Enjoy it on weekends, when you have more time to spend the night at the family table.

Ingredients :

- 2 eggs, hard

- ½ avocado

- 1 tsp olive oil

- 60 g bacon

- Salt and pepper

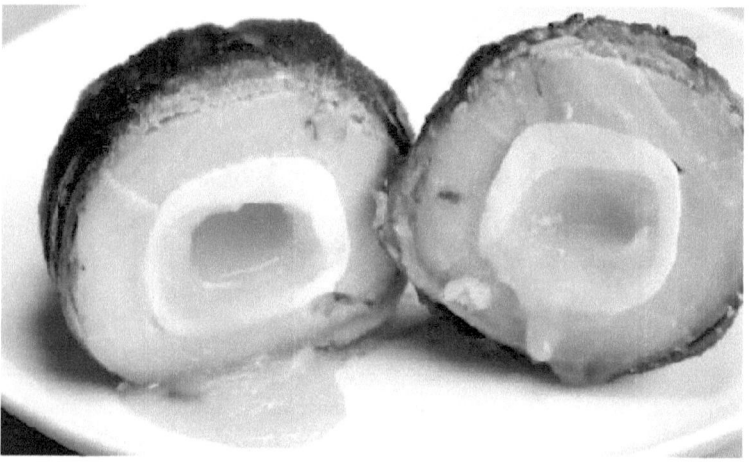

Instructions

- Preheat the oven to 180 ° C (350 ° F).

- Put the eggs in a pot and cover with water. Bring to a boil and let simmer for 8-10 minutes. Place the eggs in ice water as soon as they are made to make it easier to peel them.

- Split the eggs in two halves along and take out the yolks. Put them in a small bowl.

- Add avocado and oil to the bowl and mash until mixed. Salt and pepper to taste.

- Place the bacon in a baking sheet and bake until crispy. Take 5-7 minutes. You can also fry them in a pan.

- With a spoon, carefully add the mixture to the egg whites and place the bacon candle. To enjoy!

Advice!

No doubt fun for children, but also fun for adults ... in addition, these eggs are durable and nice enough to be your food to the basket.

- **Eggs and Vegetables Fried in Coconut Oil**

This dish makes for a great breakfast that you can enjoy every day. It's rich in protein and healthy vegetables, keeping you full for a long time.

Ingredients:

- Coconut oil

- fresh vegetables or frozen vegetable mix (carrots, cauliflower, broccoli, green beans)

- eggs

- spices

- spinach (optional).

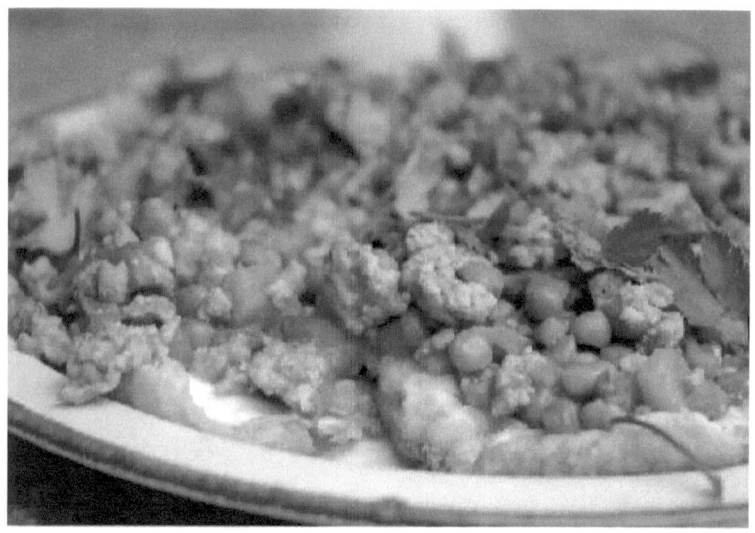

Instructions:

- Add coconut oil to your frying pan and turn up the heat.
- Add vegetables. If you use a frozen mix, let the vegetables thaw in the heat for a few minutes.
- Add 3–4 eggs.
- Add spices — either a blend or simply salt and pepper.
- Add spinach (optional).
- Stir-fry until ready.

- **Grilled Chicken Wings With Greens and Salsa**

This one may just become one of your favorites. It takes little preparation, and most people love to eat meat straight off the bone — you may even find it meets your kid's approval.

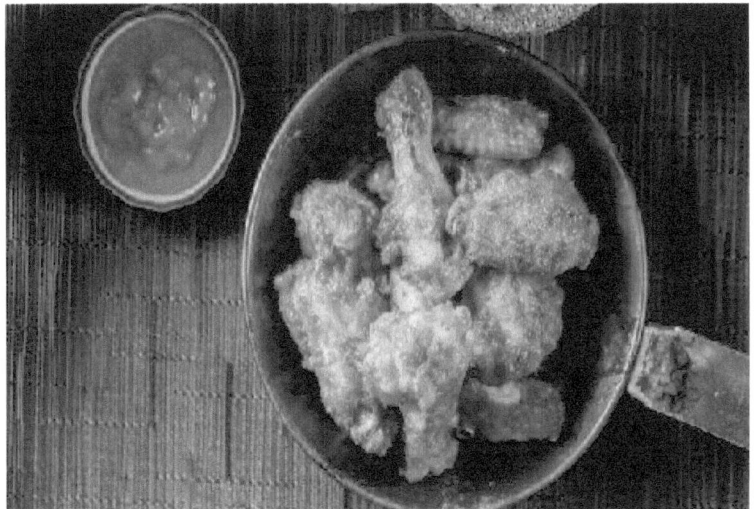

Ingredients:

- Chicken wings

- Spices

- Greens

- Salsa.

Directions :

- Rub the chicken wings in a spice blend of your choice.

- Place them in the oven and heat at 360–395°F (180–200°C) for about 40 minutes.

- Grill until the wings are brown and crunchy.

- Serve with some greens and salsa.

- **Keto Saandwich Breakfast**

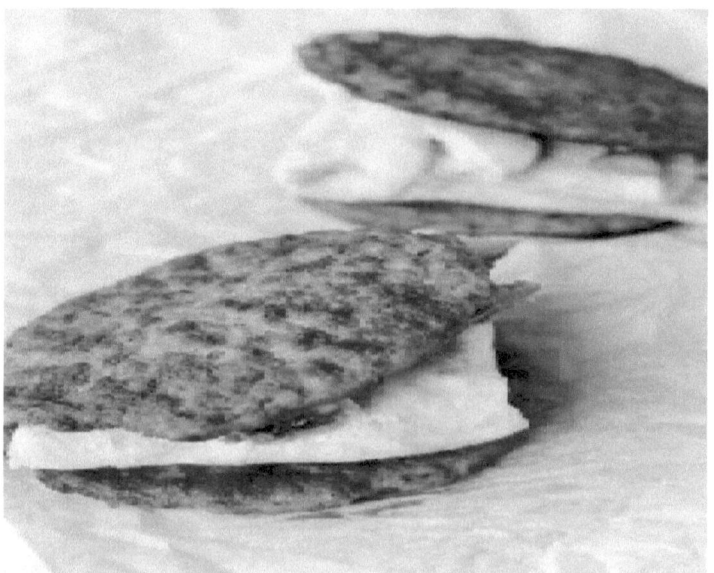

This is the Keto breakfast sandwich. High in filling healthy fats and low in carbs. You won't miss the bread because you'll be too busy loving the sausage!

Ingredients:

- 2 sausage patties

- 1 egg
- 1 tbsp cream cheese
- 2 tbsp sharp cheddar
- 1/4 medium avocado, sliced
- 1/4-1/2 tsp sriracha (to taste)
- Salt, pepper to taste

Instructions:

1. In skillet over medium heat, cook sausages per package instructions and set aside
2. In small bowl place cream cheese and sharp cheddar. Microwave for 20-30 seconds until melted
3. Mix cheese with sriracha, set aside
4. Mix egg with seasoning and make small omelette
5. Fill omelette with cheese sriracha mixture and assemble sandwich

- **Keto Chorizo Omelette**

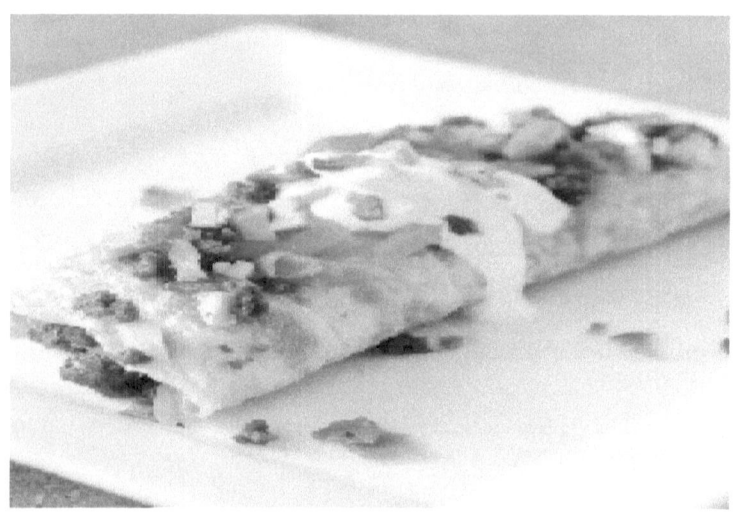

Ingredients:

- omelette
- 2 Large Eggs
- 1/4 Cup Spinach, Chopped
- 2 Tablespoons White Onion
- 2 tablespoons Heavy Whipping Cream
- 2 Ounces of Chorizo
- 1/4 Cup Cheddar Cheese, Shredded
- Salt & Pepper to Taste

Toppings:

- 1 Tablespoon Sour Cream

- 1/8 cup of diced avocado
- 1 Slice of Bacon, Crumbled

Instructions:

1. Cook Chorizo According to Package Instructions
2. In a medium bowl, whisk eggs, spinach, heavy whipping cream, and onion.
3. Pour mixture into non-stick skillet at low to medium heat
4. Flip omelette when firm enough. Cover omelette briefly with lid if not firming up
5. Sprinkle Cheese on other side and cook evenly
6. Remove from heat and place on plate
7. Add Chorizo to omelette and roll egg
8. Top with Sour Cream, Diced Avocado, Bacon and more Chorizo

- **Breakfast Pizza Frittata**

At just over 2.1 net carbs per serving, this Low Carb Breakfast Pizza makes a fabulous ketogenic breakfast or lunc,! It's delicious! Eggs, heavy cream, sausage, peppers, and cheese come together to make a super filling low carb meal!

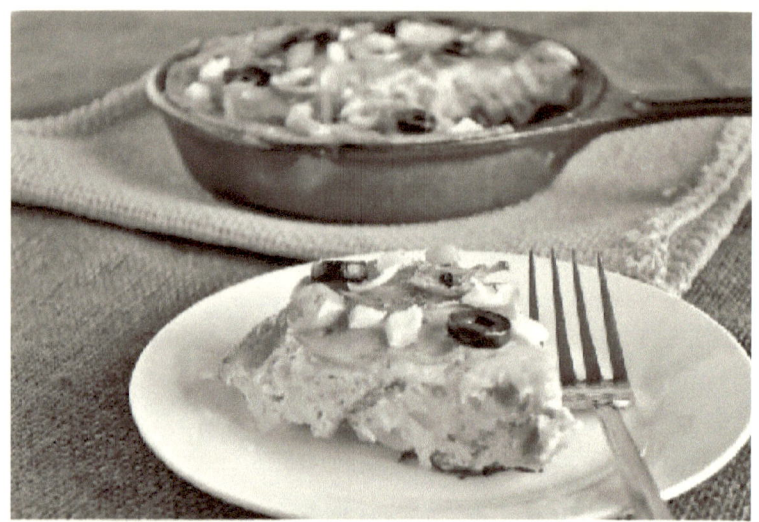

Ingredients:

- 12 eggs
- 1/2 cup heavy cream
- 1/2 teaspoon salt
- 1/4 teaspoon pepper
- 8 oz sausage
- 2 cups peppers sliced
- 1 cup cheese shredded

Instructions:

1. Preheat oven to 350 degrees.
2. Add peppers to microwave for 3 minutes.

3. Brown sausage in cast iron skillet.

4. Take out and set aside.

5. Mix eggs, cream, salt and pepper together and add to skillet.

6. Cook for 5 minutes until the sides start to set up.

7. Add to oven and bake for 15 minutes.

8. Take out and add sausage, peppers and cheese.

9. Set under broiler for 3 minutes.

10. Let sit for 5 minutes.

- **Keto Cauliflower Hash Browns**

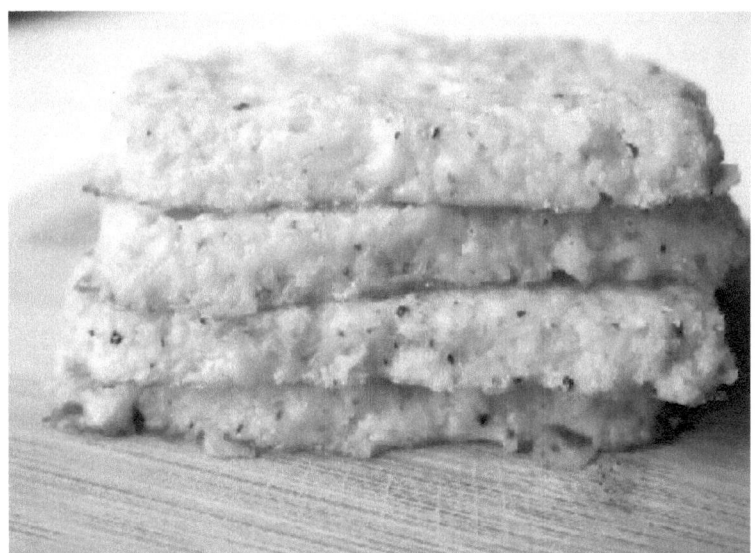

<u>**Ingredients:**</u>

- 0.17 small head grated cauliflower(about 3 cups)
- 0.17 large Egg
- 0.13 cup Shredded Cheddar Cheese
- 0.04 tsp Cayenne Pepper (optional)
- 0.04 tsp garlic powder
- 0.08 tsp Pink Salt
- 0.02 tsp black pepper

Instructions:

1. Grate entire head of cauliflower.
2. Microwave for 3 minutes and let cool. Place in paper towels or cheese cloth and ring out all the excess water.
3. Place rung out cauliflower in a bowl, add rest of ingredients and combine well.
4. Form into six square shaped hash browns on a greased baking tray.
5. Place in a 400 degree oven for 15-20 minutes.
6. Let cool for 10 minutes and hash browns will firm up. Serve warm Enjoy!

Keto Lunch Recipes

- **Taco Salad Recipe With Ground Beef**

Salad are perfect for lunch because they are extremely easy to make.The same case applies to this , super easy to make and with common ingredients. After browning the meat(the only cooking involved) all you do is mixeverything together.You can also omit anything you don't like and add other veggies as long as they are Keto Friendly.

<u>Ingredients:</u>

- 75.6 g Ground beef
- 0.82 ml Avocado oil (or any oil of choice)
- 4.93 g Taco seasoning (store-bought or home-made)
- 37.8 g Romaine lettuce (chopped)
- 33.11 g Grape tomatoes (halved)
- 14.13 g Cheddar cheese (shredded)
- 0.17 medium Avocado (cubed)
- g Scallions (chopped)
- 14.45 g Tomato salsa
- Sour cream

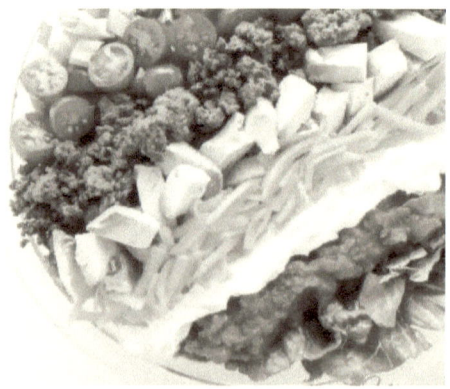

Instructions:

1. Heat oil in a skillet over high heat. Add ground beef. Stir fry, breaking up the pieces with a spatula, for about 7-10 minutes, until the beef is browned and moisture has evaporated.

2. Stir taco seasoning into the ground beef until well combined.

3. Meanwhile, combine all remaining ingredients in a large bowl. Add the ground beef. Toss everything together.

* **Low Carb Keto Cheese Taco Shells**

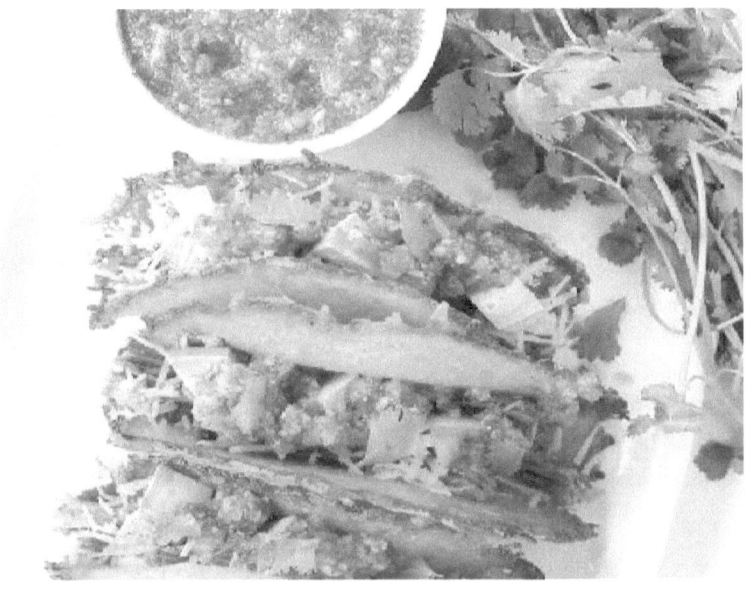

Ingredients:

- 0.67 cup Cheddar cheese (shredded)
- 0.08 tsp Cumin
- 0.04 tsp Chili powder

Instructions :

1. Preheat the oven to 375 degrees F (191 degrees C). Line either two jelly roll pans or one XL baking sheet with parchment paper.

2. Place cheese in circles on the baking sheet(s), with even thickness throughout. Sprinkle with cumin and chili powder.

3. Bake for 5-7 minutes, until the edges start to brown and bubbles start to form.

4. Meanwhile, setup wooden spoons sitting horizontally across two overturned glasses (see picture above with the cheese on it). This way, they'll be ready once the cheese taco shells are out of the oven.

5. Remove the pan(s) from the oven and cool without disturbing for about 1 minute.

6. Use a flat turner or spatula to lift the cheese circles and hang them over the wooden spoons. Let them hang until hardened, about 5 minutes.

- **Flaxseed Keto Wrap**

These flaxseed keto wraps are extremely delicious,nutritious and a better alternate to bread.The best part is that you can fill it with anything you like as long as it's keto friendly.

Servings: **2**

Ingredients:

- 1 large eggs
- 2 tbsp flax seeds milled
- 0.08 cup / 30g pre-shredded mozzarella
- 2 tbsp water
- 0.08 tsp xanthan gum optional

Instructions :

1. Mix all ingredients in a food processor or with a stick blender on a high speed until well-combined.

2. Heat butter or olive oil in a non-stick frying pan (I used an 8 inch / 20cm pan) over medium heat.

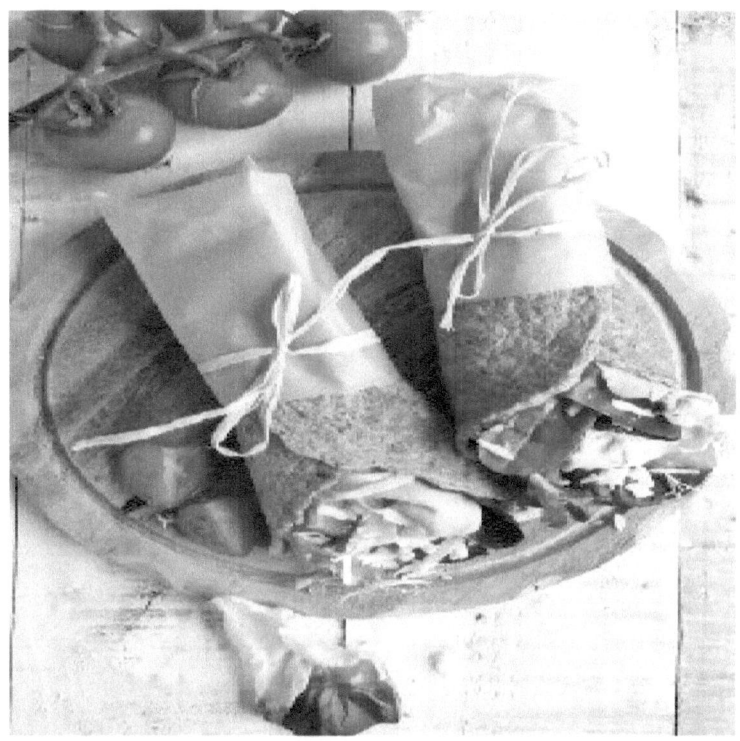

3. Scoop 2 tbsp of batter into the pan, swirl the pan around so the batter can fill the bottom of the pan. Once the top begins to bubble, flip your low carb wrap over to brown the other side.

4. Recipe Notes

5. Blend, blend, BLEND! The better your ingredients are combined, the easier it will be to fry the wraps. You don't want to end up with mozzarella clumps that take ages to melt.

6. Flaxseed has a tendency to absorb li*q*uid. If you find your batter is getting too thick towards the end of preparing your wraps, add another splash of water.

7. Medium heat works best. If you use butter to fry, clean the pan between wraps to ensure it does not burn.

8. You could customise your wraps with spices - cumin would work well, or paprika, garlic powder, onion powder or even cayenne pepper.

9. This mixture makes 2 wraps

- **Easy Keto Lasagna**

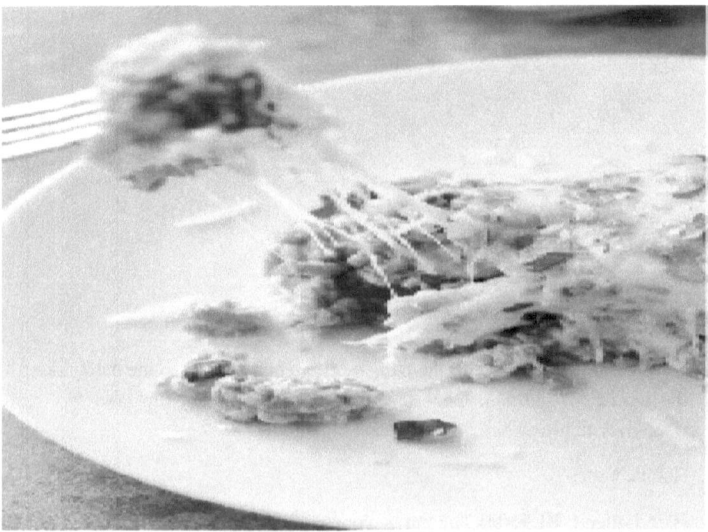

If you don't like zucchini in your lasagna then this is a recipe you will love.As with most recipes you can also tweak it a bit to suit you.It's very delicious,you will not hold yourself from going for seconds.

Servings: 6

Ingredients :

meat sauce

- 1 pound ground beef
- 1 cup raw spinach
- 1/2 cup low carb alfredo sauce
- ricotta mixture
- 1/4 cup mozzarella cheese
- 1/4 cup grated parmesan
- 1/4 cup ricotta cheese
- 3 tbsp heavy cream
- 1/2 tsp Italian seasoning

cauliflower layers

- 1 lb riced cauliflower, cooked
- 2 eggs
- 1/2 cup mozzarella
- 1/4 cup grated parmesan
- seasonings, to taste (I added garlic, salt, pepper, and Italian seasoning)

Instructions:

1. Preheat oven to 375
2. cauliflower layer
3. Grate fresh cauliflower or use prepared bag of cauliflower rice. Brown over medium heat in a skillet and drain all excess liquid using cheese cloth or towel.

4. Mix eggs, mozzarella, grated Parmesan, and seasoning in large bowl with cauliflower rice

5. Spread cauliflower rice mixture out like a pizza crust, about 1/4-1/2 inch thick on lined baking sheet

6. Bake for 15 minutes or until golden brown, set aside

7. meat sauce (while cauliflower layer bakes)

8. Brown ground beef in skillet, drain fat, and add alfredo sauce and raw spinach

9. Reduce heat and continue cooking until spinach is wilted, set aside

ricotta filling

1. Mix ricotta, grated parmesan, heavy whipping cream and seasoning together, set aside

2. assembly

3. Oven at 375

4. Prepare an 8×8 baking dish with non stick spray

5. Cut cauliflower sheet into 2 halves and trim to fit the pan

6. Place one layer of cauliflower on the bottom of the pan (I had to trim mine a little)

7. Place half of meat sauce on top of layer, adding a couple additional tsps of alfredo if needed

8. Add half of ricotta mixture on top of meat sauce layer and sprinkle 1/4 cup mozzarella

9. Place second half of cauliflower layer and repeat last two previous steps with mozzarella on top

10. Bake for 20 minutes until bubbling then broil for 3-5 minutes to brown cheese

- **Keto Grilled Lemon Herb Mediterranean Chicken Salad**

This salad will leave you wanting more.It's full of Mediterranean flavors. Olives,tomatoes,cucumbers,and avocado with olive oil. Simply mouth watering.

Servings: 4 people

Ingredients :

- Marinade/Dressing:
- 2 tablespoons olive oil
- juice of 1 lemon (1/4 cup fresh squeezed lemon juice)
- 2 tablespoons water
- 2 tablespoons red wine vinegar
- 2 tablespoons fresh chopped parsley
- 2 teaspoons dried basil
- 2 teaspoons garlic , minced

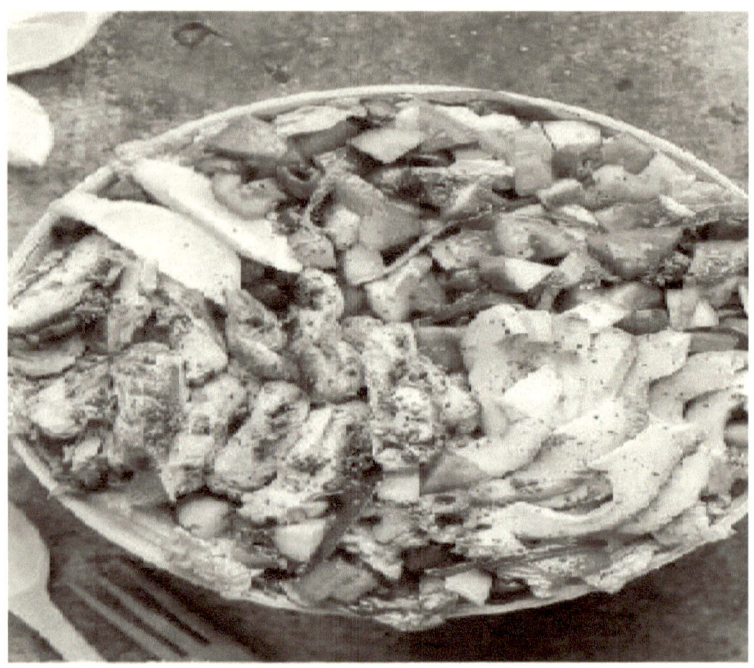

- 1 teaspoon dried oregano

- 1 teaspoon salt

- cracked pepper , to taste

- 1 pound (500 g) skinless, boneless chicken thigh fillets (or chicken breasts)

- Salad:

- 4 cups Romaine (or Cos) lettuce leaves, washed and dried

- 1 large cucumber diced

- 2 Roma tomatoes diced

- 1 red onion sliced

- 1 avocado sliced

- 1/3 cup pitted Kalamata olives (or black olives), sliced (optional)

- Lemon wedges to serve

Instructions :

1. Whisk together all of the marinade/dressing ingredients in a large jug. Pour out half of the marinade into a large, shallow dish. Refrigerate the remaining marinade to use as the dressing later.

2. Add the chicken to the marinade in the bowl; marinade chicken for 15-30 minutes (or up to two hours in the refrigerator if time allows). While waiting for the chicken, prepare all of the salad ingredients and mix in a large salad bowl.

3. Once chicken is ready, heat 1 tablespoon of oil in a grill pan or a grill plate over medium-high heat. Grill chicken on both sides until browned and completely cooked through.

4. Allow chicken to rest for 5 minutes; slice and arrange over salad. Drizzle salad with the remaining untouched dressing. Serve with lemon wedges.

- **Keto Mexican Cauliflower Rice**

This is a savory dish and it compliments any low carb mexican dish so well. As with any mexican dish this one is extremely flavourable and sastisfying too.Especially if you've been struggling to make cauliflower rice a part of your diet, you need to try this recipe!

Serving : 4

Ingredients :

- 4 cups fresh riced cauliflower (about 1 medium head)

- 2 tablespoons coconut oil

- 2 tablespoons tomato paste

- 1/4 cup onion, chopped

- 1 small jalapeno, chopped

- 1 clove garlic, minced

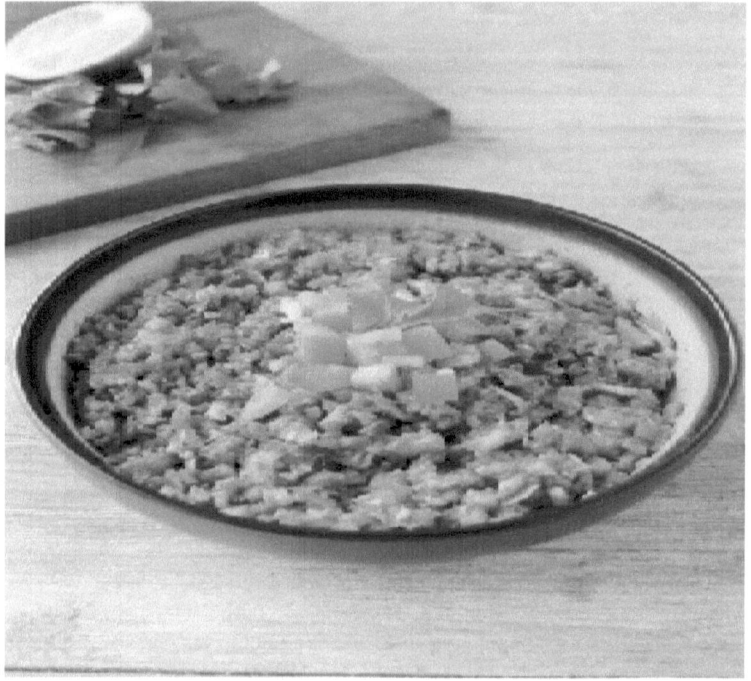

- 1/2 cup chicken broth

- 1 teaspoon chili powder

- salt & pepper, to taste

- 1/4 cup cilantro, chopped

- diced tomato, optional
- sour cream, optional

Instructions:

1. Remove core and leaves from cauliflower. Cut into florets and pulse in food processor or use grater. Set aside.

2. In skillet, over medium heat, add coconut oil and tomato paste. As coconut oil melts, gently mix with tomato paste.

3. Add onion and jalapeno to pan. Cook until the mixture begins to soften, about 3-5 minutes.

4. Add garlic to pan and sir for 30 seconds, then pour in chicken broth.

5. Add riced cauliflower to pan. Sprinkle salt and chili powder over cauliflower and gently fold into broth until coated and red.

6. Continue cooking cauliflower until most moisture in the pan has evaporated and cauliflower is tender, about 10-15 minutes.

7. Turn off heat and fold in cilantro. Serve with diced tomatoes, sour cream, and additional cilantro, if desired.

Notes : You can use frozen cauliflower, but you may need to reduce the amount of broth.

- **Keto Chicken Enchilada Bowl**

Servings : 4

Ingredients :

- 2 tablespoons coconut oil (for searing chicken)
- 1 pound of boneless, skinless chicken thighs
- 3/4 cup red enchilada sauce (recipe from Low Carb Maven)

- 1/4 cup water
- 1/4 cup chopped onion
- 1– 4 oz can diced green chiles
- toppings (feel free to customize)
- 1 whole avocado, diced

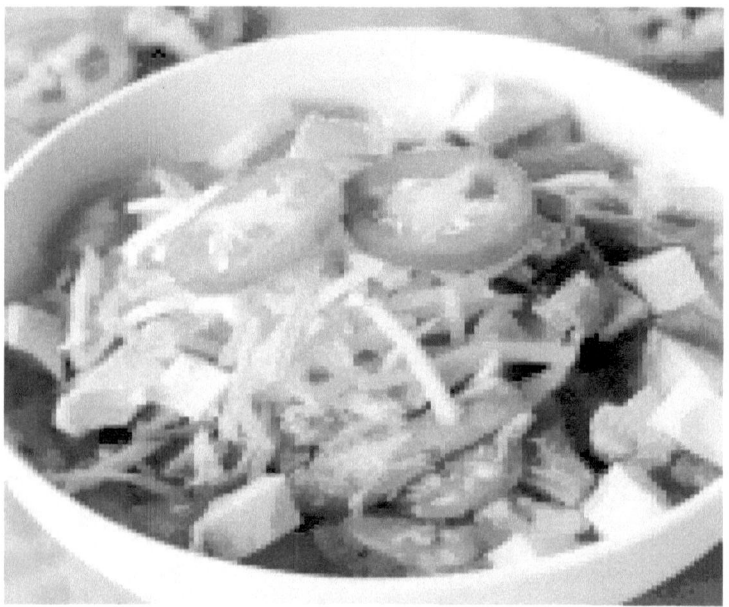

- 1 cup shredded cheese (you can use mild cheddar)
- 1/4 cup chopped pickled jalapenos
- 1/2 cup sour cream
- 1 roma tomato, chopped

Optional: serve over plain cauliflower rice (or mexican cauliflower rice) for a more complete meal!

Instructions :

1. In a pot or dutch oven over medium heat melt the coconut oil. Once hot, sear chicken thighs until lightly brown.

2. Pour in enchilada sauce and water then add onion and green chiles. Reduce heat to a simmer and cover. Cook chicken for 17-25 minutes or until chicken is tender and fully cooked through to at least 165 degrees internal temperature.

3. Careully remove the chicken and place onto a work surface. Chop or shred chicken (your preference) then add it back into the pot. Let the chicken simmer uncovered for an additional 10 minutes to absorb flavor and allow the sauce to reduce a little.

4. To Serve, top with avocado, cheese, jalapeno, sour cream, tomato, and any other desired toppings. Feel free to customize these to your preference. Serve alone or over cauliflower rice if desired just be sure to update your personal nutrition info as needed.

- **Loaded Keto Cauliflower Bowl**

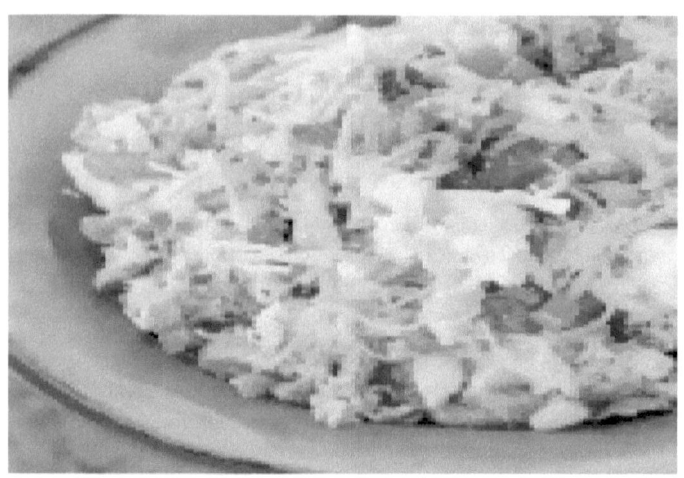

Servings: 4

Ingredients :

- 2 cups fresh cauliflower
- 3 tablespoons butter
- ¼ cup diced onion
- ¼ cup pickled jalapeno slices
- 2 cups cooked brisket
- 2 ounces cream cheese, softened
- 1 cup shredded sharp cheddar
- ¼ cup heavy cream
- ¼ cup cooked crumbled bacon
- 2 tablespoons sliced green onions

Instructions :

1. Chop cauliflower into bite size pieces. Steam or cook via favorite method until fork tender and set side.

2. Set heat to medium and add butter, onion, and jalapeno slices to skillet. Saute until onions translucent and fragrant.

3. Reduce heat slightly and add cooked brisket [or choice of leftover beef/ chicken] and cream cheese.If mixture begins to stick or cook too quickly, reduce heat a bit. Continue cooking until cream cheese is heated through and easily stirred.

4. Turn off heat. Add sharp cheddar, heavy cream and cauliflower. Stir mixture quickly until all cheeses are melted and fully combined.

5. Sprinkle with crumbled bacon, green onions. Serve warm.

6. notes

7. Feel free to substitute chicken or other shredded beef as your meat.

- **Balsamic Avocado Bowls**

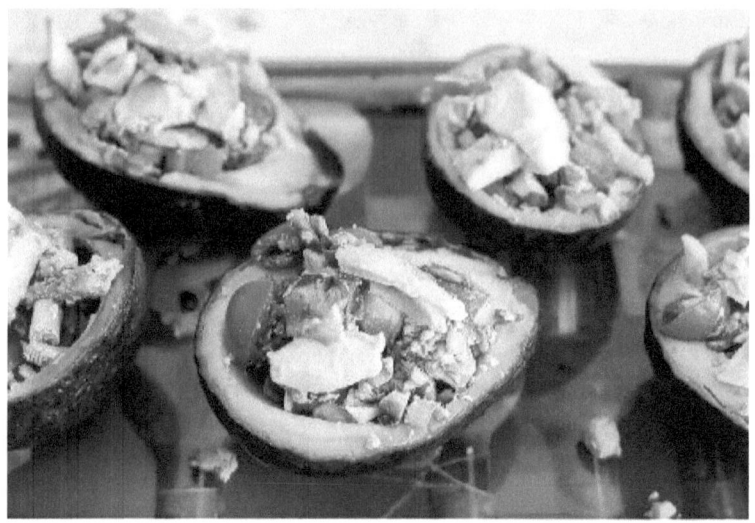

For this recipe, you can use a little liquid smoke to add some extra flavor to the cheese. If you don't have the smoke, you can always skip it then add the cheese without heating it first. If you like things spicy, then you can make this recipe hotter with Sriracha or chili flakes.

Ingredients:

- 3 medium avocados, halved

- 50 grams mushrooms, chopped

- 1 medium green onion, chopped

- 10 cherry tomatoes, chopped

- 45 grams goat cheese, crumbled

- 1 tablespoon olive oil

- 1 tablespoon liquid smoke
- ½ teaspoon paprika
- 3 tablespoons balsamic vinegar

Directions :

1. Preheat a frying pan over medium heat. Add mushrooms, green onions, and tomatoes into a mixing bowl.

2. Heat the olive oil, liquid smoke, and paprika in the pan.

3. Add in the goat cheese.

4. Saute until the cheese is nicely browned.

5. Remove the pan from the stove. Add goat cheese into the mixing bowl. Mix together.

6. Scoop out a small portion of flesh from inside the avocado halves to create enough room for the filling. Set aside the scooped out avocado.

7. Spoon the salad mix into the avocado shells. Garnish with the scooped out avocado. Pour a half teaspoon of balsamic vinegar onto each.

- **Keto Cauliflower Tabboule**

This makes a total of 6 (½-cup) servings of Keto Cauliflower Tabbouleh. Each serving comes out to be 158.72 Calories, 14.52g Fat, 3.82g Net Carbs, and 2.47g Protein.

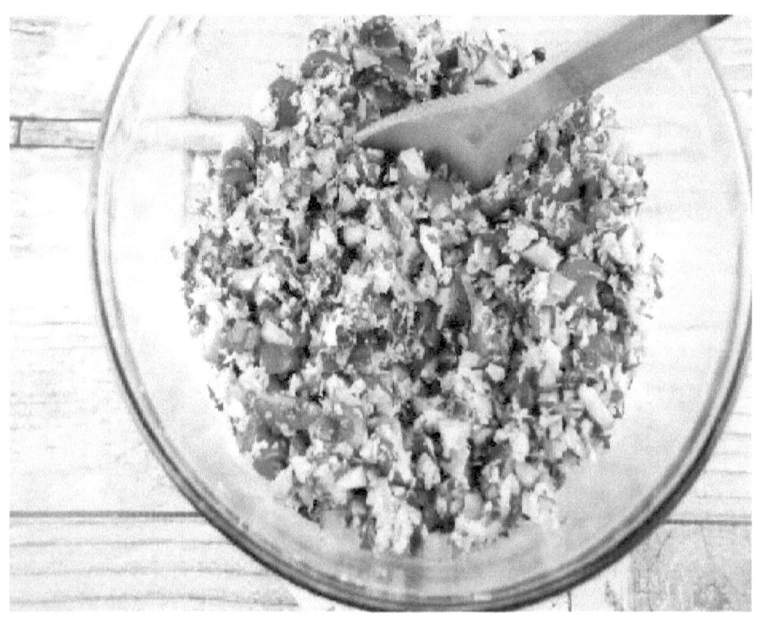

Ingredients:

- 1 1/2 cups riced cauliflower
- 1/4 cup chopped red onion
- 1/4 cup diced red bell pepper
- 1/2 cup diced cucumber
- 12 large Kalamata Olives
- 1/4 cup lemon juice
- 1/4 cup olive oil
- Salt and Pepper, to taste

- 1 cup chopped parsley
- 1 cup chopped mint leaves
- 1/2 medium avocado, diced
- 1 ounce slivered almonds

Directions :

- In a large bowl, combine the riced cauliflower, red onion, bell pepper, cucumber and Kalamata olives.
- Drizzle the veggies in the lemon juice and olive oil. Season with salt and pepper and stir to coat.
- Fold in chopped parsley and mint.
- Add diced avocado to the bowl and gently mix in.
- Top with slivered almonds. Serve chilled.

- **Keto Taco Salad**

Ingredients :

- ¾ pound ground beef
- 1 teaspoon ground cumin
- ½ teaspoon chili powder
- 1 teaspoon dried parsley
- 1 teaspoon garlic powder

- 8 ounces romaine lettuce, chopped

- 9 ounces iceberg lettuce, chopped

- 2 small red tomatoes, chopped

- 1 ½ cups pre-shredded mozzarella cheese

- 1 medium avocado, chopped

- 1 cup sour cream

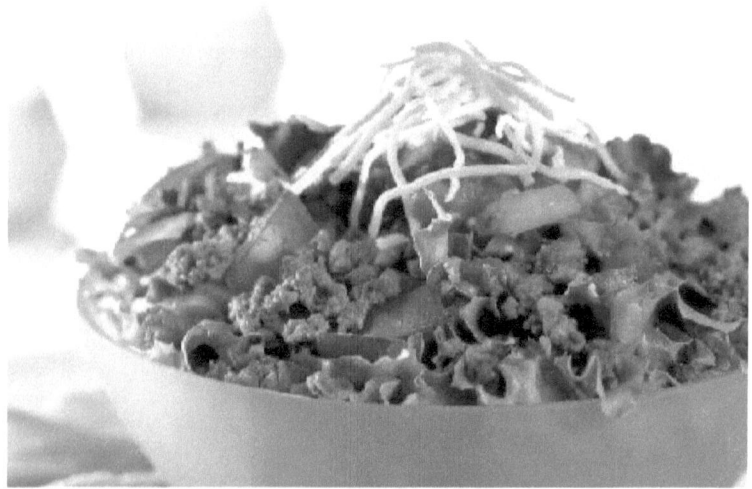

Directions:

- Pre-heat a non-stick pan on a stove. Put ground beef into the pan.

- Place herbs and spices on ground beef. Cook ground beef on medium heat. Once it's done remove the pan from the stove. Allow ground beef to drain and cool. Set aside.

- Place chopped lettuce, tomatoes, shredded mozzarella, and avocado into a salad bowl. Mix salad ingredients well.

- Top the salad mix with ground beef and sour cream.

• **Maple Shrimp Salad**

Maple Shrimp Salad is a sweet and savory dish that can be served as a side salad for dinner .

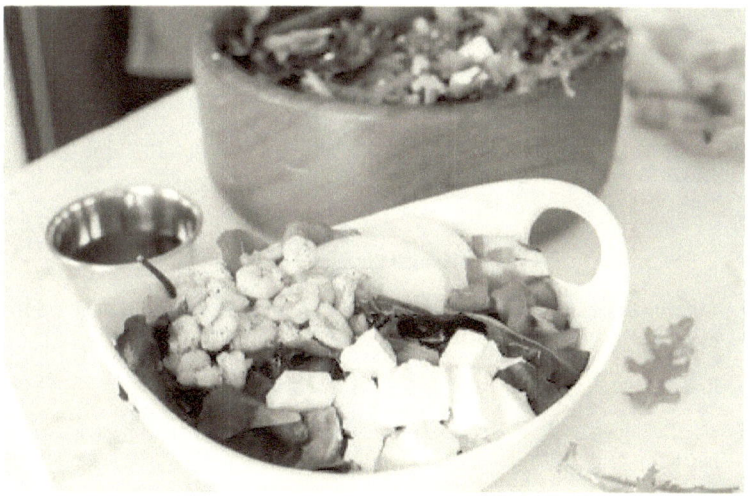

Ingredients :

- 6 ounces field greens
- 1 pound feta cheese, chopped
- 2 tablespoons butter
- 1 teaspoon minced garlic
- 2 pounds shrimp
- ½ medium onion, chopped
- 2 medium red peppers, sliced
- 3 teaspoons olive oil
- 5 teaspoons sugar-free maple syrup
- 2 teaspoons apple cider vinegar
- 1 tablespoon lemon juice

Directions :

- Pre-heat a pan on the stove then melt the butter.
- Add minced garlic to melted butter. Place shrimp in pan. Saute until lightly browned.
- Remove the pan from the stove and allow the shrimp to cool.
- Mix field greens, shrimp, chopped feta , onion, and sliced red peppers in a salad bowl.
- In a separate bowl, whisk together olive oil, sugar-free maple syrup, apple cider vinegar, and lemon juice.

- Pour salad dressing onto salad. Toss so ingredients are evenly coated.

- **Keto Coconut Flour Pizza Crust**

<u>serves : 8</u>

<u>Ingredients:</u>

- 1/3 cup coconut flour about 44 grams

- 1/4 cup parmesan cheese about 26 grams

- 2 tablespoons flaxseed meal or almond flour or psyllium

- 4 large eggs

- 1-2 tablespoon olive oil

- 1 teaspoon garlic powder

- 1/4 teaspoon salt

- 1/4 teaspoon cream of tartar

- 1 teaspoon Italian Seasoning Blend

- 1 teaspoon parsley

- 3/4 cup mozzarella cheese about 78 grams

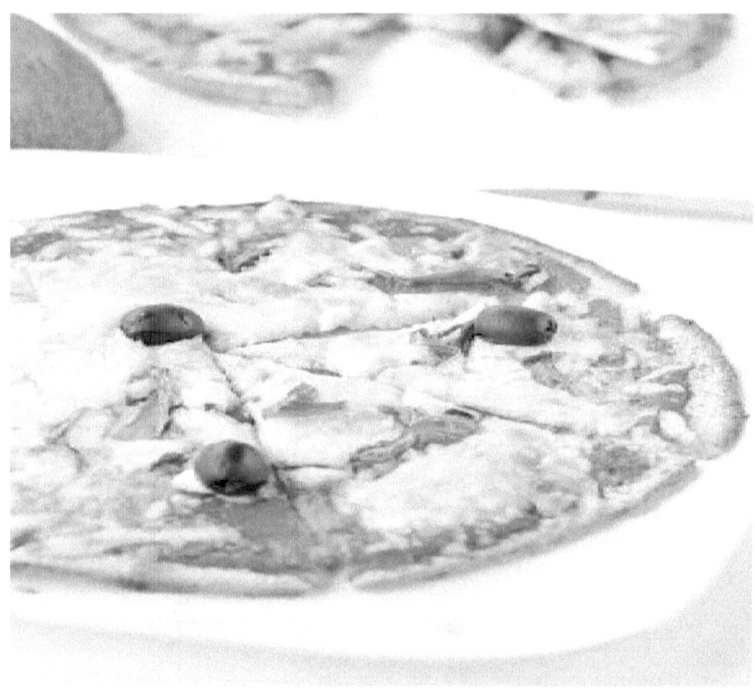

Instructions :

- Place all ingredients except mozzarella cheese into a food processor.

- Process until there are no more lumps.

- Fold in mozzarella cheese.

- Spread onto greased baking sheet or line sheet with non-stick silicon mat. Bake at 375 F for about 20-25 minutes or until top is browned.

- Slice into strips for bread sticks. For pizza, top with sauce and toppings then bake at 350 F for about 12 minutes.

- **keto buffalo chicken tenders**

<u>Yield: 4 servings</u>

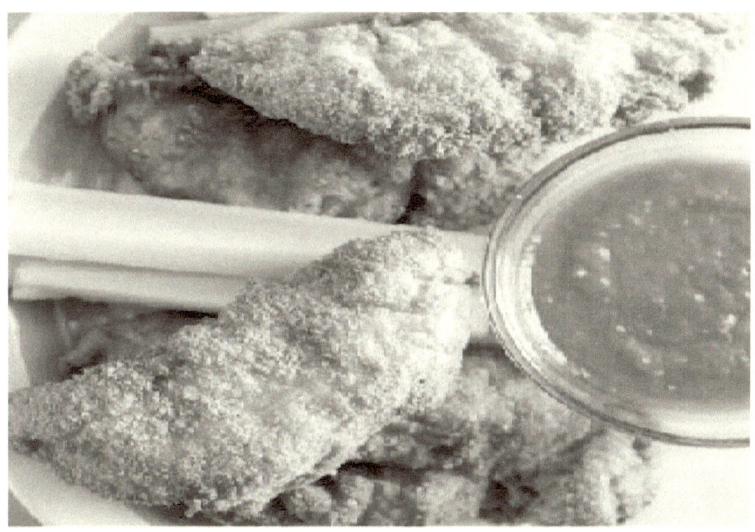

<u>INGREDIENTS :</u>

- 2 cups crushed pork rinds (get them here)
- 3/4 cup finely grated Parmesan cheese
- 1 teaspoon garlic powder
- 1 teaspoon Italian seasoning

- 1 teaspoon onion powder
- 2 large eggs
- 1 1/2 pounds boneless skinless chicken breasts, cut into tender-size pieces
- 1 cup buffalo wing sauce (I use this brand)
- 1/4 cup butter (1/2 stick)

INSTRUCTIONS :

- Combine the pork rinds, Parmesan cheese, garlic powder, Italian seasoning and onion powder and mix until well incorporated. Pour the mixture into a thin layer on a large plate.
- Crack the eggs into a shallow bowl and fork whisk. Dip the chicken tenders in the egg wash, and then dredge them in the breading mixture. Make sure both sides are thoroughly coated in the breading mixture.
- Heat 1 to 2 inches of oil is a high-sided skillet. You can use avocado oil for this. Once the oil is hot and begins to bubble slightly, drop the breaded chicken tenders into the oil. Fry until they are golden brown and crispy on both sides, about 3 minutes each side. Be careful not to flip them too much or else the breading will fall off.
- Remove the chicken tenders from the oil and place them on paper towels to absorb the excess grease.
- In a small sauce pan, heat the buffalo wing sauce and the butter over medium heat. Cook until the butter is melted and mixed into the sauce. Transfer the sauce to a large mixing bowl. Toss the tenders in the sauce until thoroughly coated.

Keto Snacks Recipes

- **Cinnamon Keto Granola**

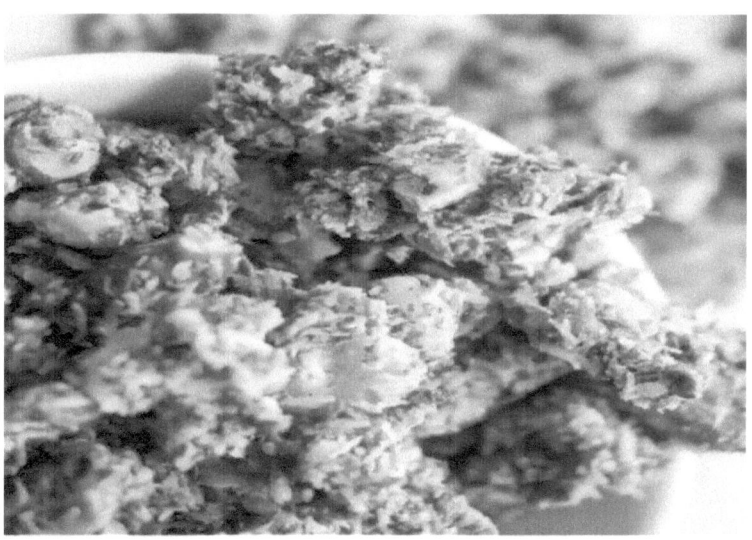

Servings 20

Ingredients:

- 5 tbsp flax seed meal
- 5 tbsp unsweetened coconut flakes
- 1 tbsp Chia Seeds
- 1.5 oz nuts (we used pecans, walnuts and almonds)

- 4 tbsp sugar free maple syrup
- 1 1/2 tsp ground cinnamon Optional

Instructions :

1. Combine all ingredients thoroughly except for the cinnamon.
2. Spread out mixture onto a baking sheet to make one layer.
3. Sprinkle on cinnamon.
4. Bake in 350 degree over for 20-22 minutes.
5. Let rest. Granola will harden as it cools. Enjoy!

- **Avocado & Egg Fat Bombs and Deviled Eggs**

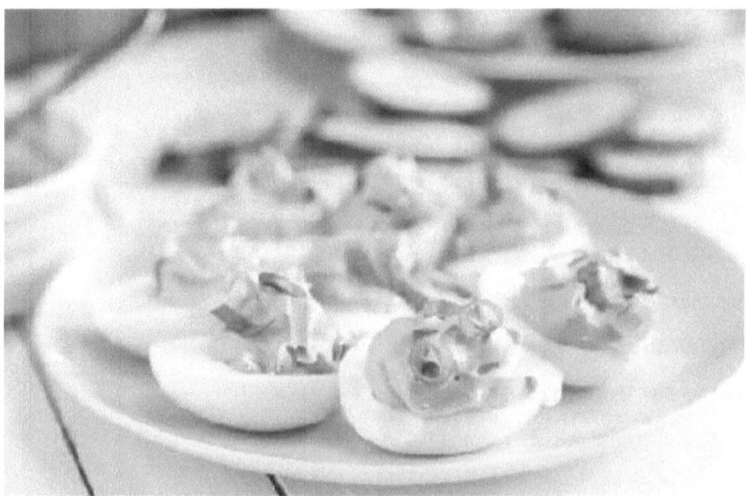

Ingredients:

- 3 large cooked egg yolks
- 1/2 large avocado, peeled and seed removed (100 g/ 3.5 oz)
- 1/4 cup mayonnaise (55 g/ 1.9 oz) - you can make your own
- 1 tbsp lemon or lime juice
- 1/2 tsp salt or to taste .
- freshly ground black pepper
- 2 tbsp chopped spring onions or chives

Eat with:

- freshly cut cucumber slices, bell peppers or crispy lettuce leaves
- leftover cooked egg white halves (if making deviled eggs)

Instructions :

1. Start by cooking the eggs. Fill a small saucepan with water up to three quarters. Add a good pinch of salt. This will prevent the eggs from cracking. Bring to a boil. Using a spoon or hand, dip each egg in and out of the boiling water - be careful not to get burnt. This will prevent the egg from cracking as the temperature change won't be so sudden. To get the eggs hard-boiled, you need round 10 minutes. This timing works for large eggs. When done, remove from the heat and place in a bowl filled with cold water. You can use egg timer! When the eggs are chilled, peel off the shells.

2. Halve the avocado and remove the seed and peel. Cut the eggs in half and carefully - without breaking the egg whites - spoon the egg yolks into a bowl.

3. Place the avocado cut into pieces into a food processor and add the egg yolks, mayonnaise, lemon juice, salt and pepper. Process until smooth. Alternatively, mash with a fork until creamy and well combined.

4. Enjoy with cucumber slices and spring onion on top, or ...... fill up the egg white halves and make deviled eggs. To avoid browning, store in an airtight container and keep for up to 5 days.

- **Salt & Vinegar Zucchini Chips**

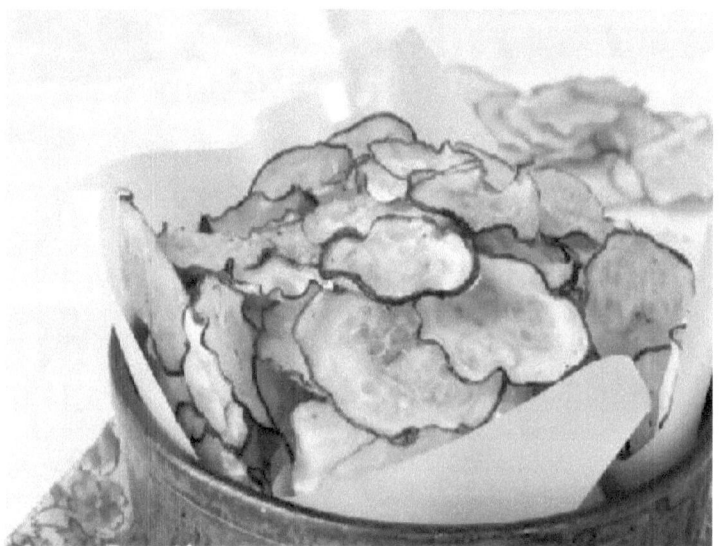

Ingredients:

- 4 cups thinly sliced zucchini about 2-3 medium
- 2 tablespoons extra virgin olive oil avocado oil or sunflower oil
- 2 tablespoons white balsamic vinegar
- 2 teaspoons coarse sea salt

Instructions:

1. Use a mandolin or slice zucchini as thin as possible.

2. In a small bowl whisk olive oil and vinegar together.

3. Place zucchini in a large bowl and toss with oil and vinegar.

4. Add zucchini in even layers to dehydrator then sprinkle with coarse sea salt.

5. Depending on how thin you sliced the zucchini and on your dehydrator the drying time will vary, anywhere from 8-14 hours. My temperature setting was 135 degrees F.

6. To make in the oven: Line a cookie sheet with parchment paper. Lay zucchini evenly. Bake at 200 degrees F for 2-3 hours. Rotate half way during cooking time.

7. Store chips in an airtight container.

- **Quick And Easy Antipasto Skewers**

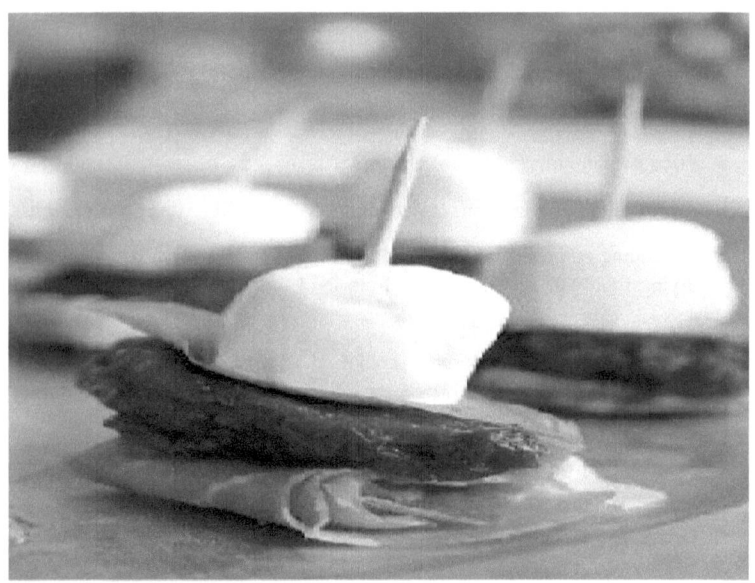

Servings: 30

Ingredients :

- 8 Prosciutto , slices
- 16 Ciliegine (1 inch) mozzarella balls
- 16 Sun dried tomatoes , in oil
- 16 Basil leaves

Instructions :

1. Cut prosciutto slices in half.

2. Fold up prosciutto and place one sun dried tomato, one basil leaf, and one mozzarella ball on top of it.

3. Skewer with a toothpick.

4. 5.Cheese Stuffed Jalapeno Peppers

- **Stuffed Jalapeno**

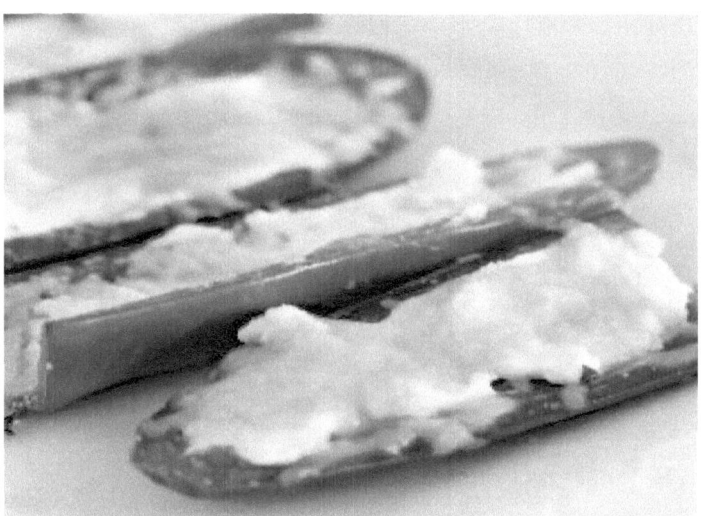

Ingredients :

- 15 Fresh whole jalapenos
- 8 oz package of cream cheese
- 8 oz shredded cheese (Cheddar or colby jack)
- Garlic salt

Optional: You could add browned sausage or crumbled up bacon if you want for a new twist.

Instructions:

1. Take your whole jalapenos and slice off the stem. Then cut in half and pull out seeds (using a spoon is the fastest method). Do this for all the jalapenos you are using.

2. Place them all in a pot of water. Bring to a boil, and let boil for about 5 minutes. (This helps remove some of the heat from the pepper)

3. Drain and place all peppers (cute side up on a cookie sheet)

4. Spoon in cream cheese into each pepper.

5. Sprinkle with garlic salt and top with shredded cheese.

6. Place under broiler until brown (about 2 minutes).

7. Let set for a few minutes and then serve.

- **Keto Friendly Cheese Crackers**

Servings: 35

Ingredients :

- Cracker Sized Deli Cheese Slices – you can use Aged Cheddar French-Swiss, DutchGouda, and Havarti

- 3/4 tsp Red Pepper Flakes

- 1/4 tsp paprika

- 1/4 tsp garlic powder

Instructions:

1. Preheat oven to 325 degrees.

2. Cover cookie sheet with parchment paper.

3. Lay cheese slices flat to fill the cookie sheet. Leave a little bit of room between each slice. If they melt together it is no big deal as once they cool they will break apart easily. I used precut slices, but you can buy larger deli slices and cut them into smaller squares.

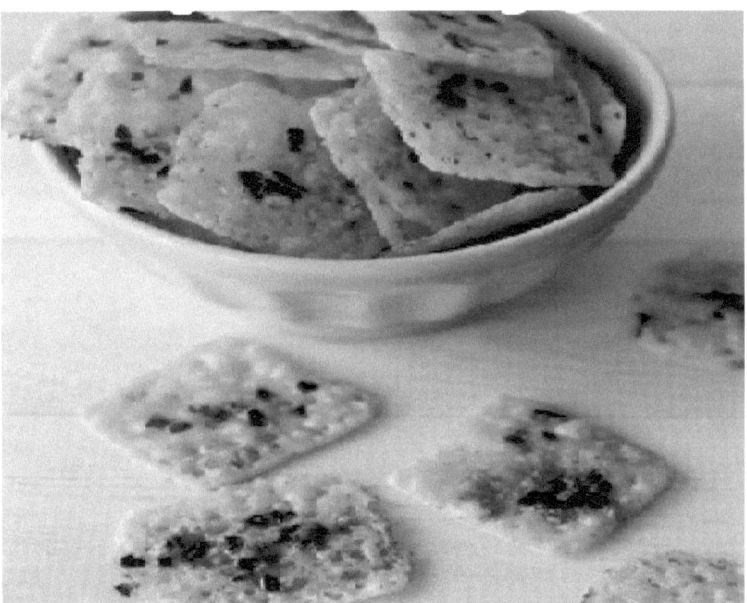

4. Sprinkle spices on cheese slices.

5. Bake for 23 minutes.

6. Remove from oven and allow to cool for 5 minutes before eating. Once they cool you can easily break apart any cheese slices that have melted together.

Note: Baking time may vary due to variances in ovens and thickness of cheese. If the cheese isn't crunchy at 23 minutes, bake a little longer

- **Turkey Bacon Ranch Pinwheels**

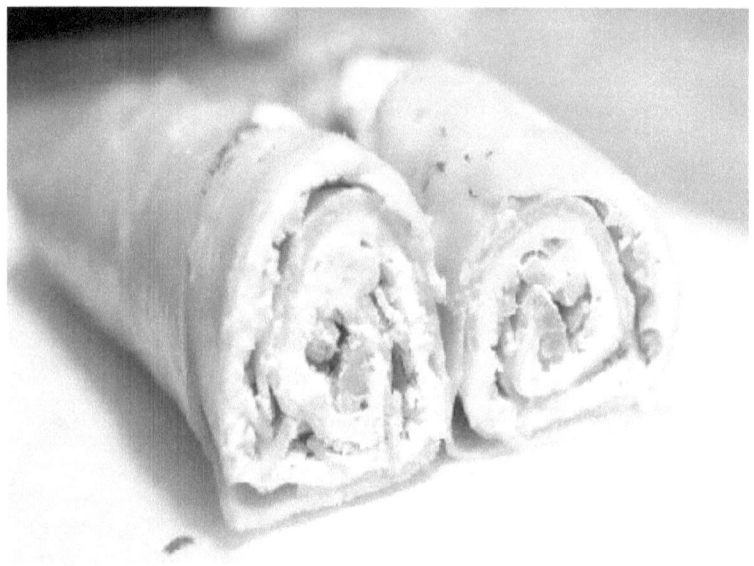

Servings 6

Ingredients:

- 6 oz cream cheese
- 12 slices smoked deli turkey about 3 oz
- 1/4 tsp each garlic powder dill, and minced onion
- 1 tbsp bacon crumbles
- 2 tbsp finely shredded cheddar cheese

Instructions:

1. Put the cream cheese between 2 pieces of plastic wrap. Roll it out until it's about 1/4 inch thick. Peel off the top piece of plastic wrap. Lay the slices of turkey on top of the cream cheese.

2. Cover with a new piece of plastic wrap and flip the whole thing over. Peel off the piece of plastic that is now on the top. Sprinkle the spices on top of the cream cheese. Sprinkle with the bacon and cheese.

3. Roll up the pinwheels so that the turkey is on the outside. Refrigerate for at least 2 hours. Thinly slice and serve on top of low carb crackers or sliced cucumber.

- **Tuna In Cucumber Cups**

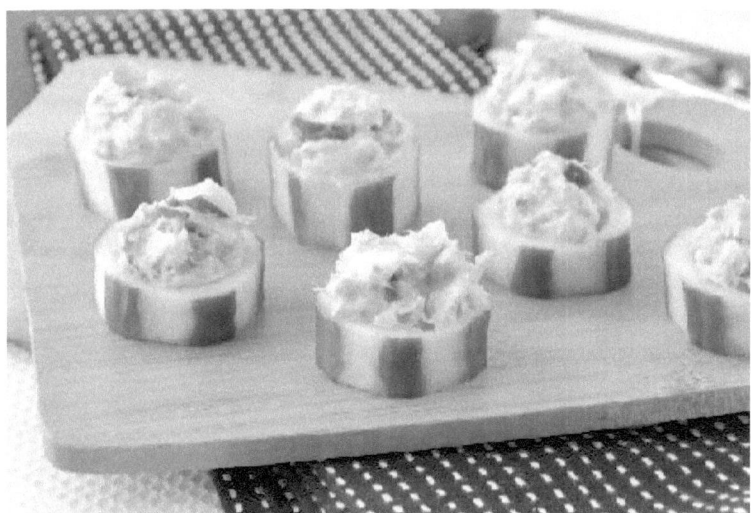

Ingredients :

- 1 large english cucumber, cut into 1" thick slices

- 1 5oz can Bumble Bee Solid White Albacore In Water tuna, drained and water squeezed out

- 1/3 cup of mayonnaise

- 1 teaspoon black pepper
- fresh dill for garnish

Instructions:

1. Using a melon baller or small spoon, scoop the seeds out of the cucumber slices, leaving about 1/4″ on the bottom to make them into little cups. Once they have all been scooped, squeeze the water from the cucumber pulp you have scooped out, and finely chop it.

2. In a small mixing bowl, combine the drained tuna, finely chopped cucumber pulp, mayo and pepper. Stir to combine. Taste to see if you want to add more mayo or pepper.

3. If your cucumber cups have a lot of moisture, dab away the water using a paper towel. Then fill each cucumber cup with tuna, and garnish with dill.

Keto Dessert Recipes

- **Keto Chocolate Roll Cake**

Ingredients :

- Chocolate Roll Cake
- 1 cup Almond Flour
- 4 tbsp. Butter, melted
- 3 large Eggs
- 1/4 cup Psyllium Husk Powder
- 1/4 cup Cocoa Powder

- 1/4 cup Coconut Milk
- 1/4 cup Sour Cream
- 1/4 cup Erythritol
- 1 tsp. Vanilla

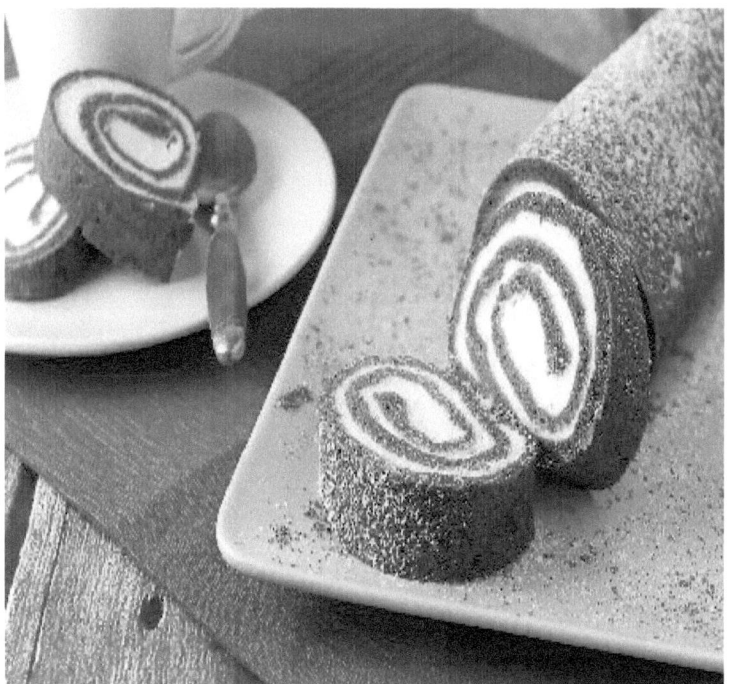

- 1 tsp. Baking Powder
- Cream Cheese Filling
- 8 oz. Cream Cheese
- 8 tbsp. Butter

- 1/4 cup Sour Cream
- 1/4 cup Erythritol
- 1/4 tsp. Stevia
- 1 tsp. Vanilla

Intructions :

1. Combine dry cake ingredients in a bowl, then slowly mix as you add the wet ingredients.
2. Spread dough on a silpat on a cookie sheet. Then bake for 12-15 minutes at 350F.
3. Let cake cook, then cream together all of the cream cheese filling ingredients.
4. Spread filling over cake, then roll cake tightly.

- **Keto coffee with cinnamon**

This hot ketogenic drink is perfect for the period of the holidays. It can even be served as a dessert.

Ingredients :

- 2 tbsp ground coffee
- 1 tsp ground cinnamon
- 475 ml water
- 75 ml whipping cream

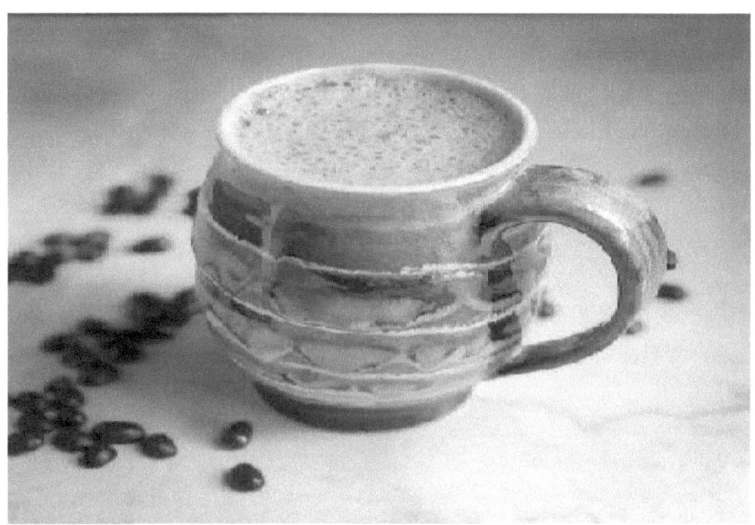

-

<u>Instructions</u>

- Mix the coffee beans with the cinnamon. Add the water and prepare the coffee in the same way you always do.

- Beat the cream by hand or with an electric mixer until it is about to firm snow.

- Serve the coffee in a nice big cup and add the whipped cream on top. Sprinkle ground cinnamon on the cream as a final touch.

- **Keto cheese cake with blueberries**

 Making a perfect keto cheese cake is easier than you think. It is sugar free and gluten free, but it still tastes great. A rich and comforting creaminess, topped with juicy fresh blueberries.

Ingredients :

- Cortex

- 300 ml (150 g) ground almonds

- 50 g butter

- 2 tbsp (25 g) erythritol

- ½ tsp. vanilla extract

- 600 g (600 ml) cream cheese

- 125 ml whipping cream or fresh cream

- 2 eggs

- 1 egg yolk

- 1 tbsp (10 g) erythritol (optional)

- 1 tsp lemons, zest

- 50 g fresh blueberries (optional)

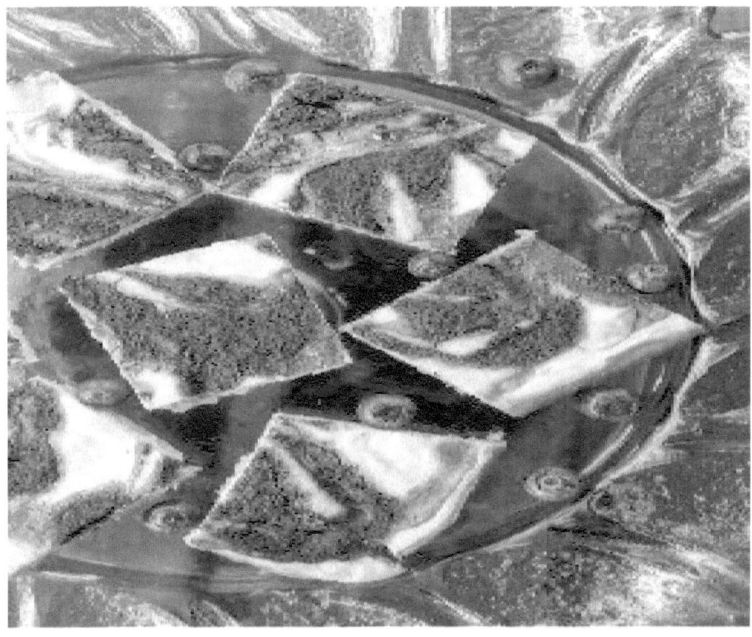

Instructions :

- Preheat the oven to 175 ° C (350 ° F). Butter a removable 22 cm (9 inch) mold with butter and line the base with baking paper.

- Melt the butter for the crust and heat until you get a scent of nuts. This will give the dough a delicious caramelized flavor.

- Remove from heat and add the almond flour, sweetener and vanilla. Mix until a dough is made and press towards the base of the removable mold. Bake for 8 minutes, until the crust browns slightly. Reserve and let cool while you prepare the filling.

- Mix cream cheese, whipping cream, eggs, lemon zest, vanilla and sweetener if you are using any. Mix well. Pour the mixture over the crust.

- Turn the heat to 200 ° C (400 ° F) and bake for 15 minutes.

- Lower the heat to 110 ° C (230 ° F) and bake for another 45-60 minutes.

- Turn off the heat and let cool in the oven. Remove when it has cooled completely and place it in the refrigerator so that it rests overnight. Serve with fresh blueberries.

* **Ketogenic bacon and cheddar cheese balls**

These balls of bacon and cheese are not only fantastic: they are ketotatics! Smoked bacon and cheddar cheese matured together produce a wonderful combination of flavors. You will only have to look at the astonished face of your guests when you serve them to know that this dish is really something else.

Ingredients

- 150 g bacon

- 1 tbsp Butter

- 150 g (150 ml) cream cheese

- 150 g cheddar cheese

- 50 g butter, at room temperature

- ½ tsp. ground black pepper (optional)

- ½ tsp. Chili flakes (optional)

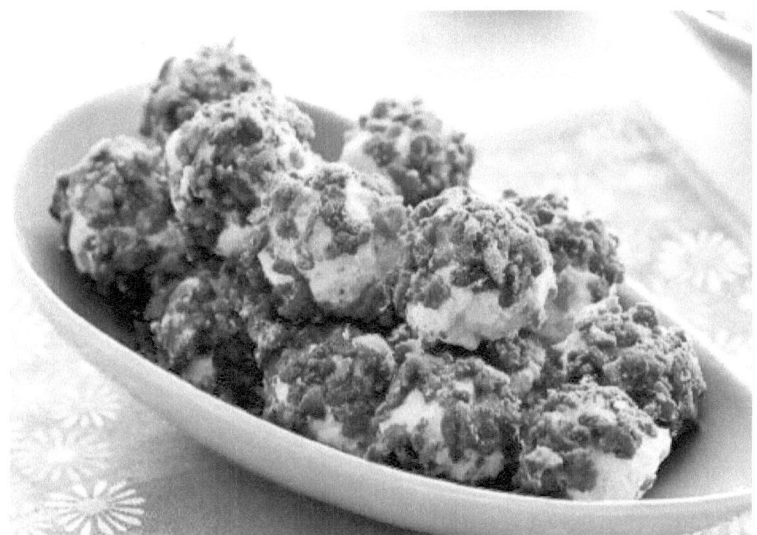

Instructions

- Fry the bacon in butter until golden brown. Take it out of the pan and let it cool completely on some absorbent papers.

- Chop or chop the bacon into small pieces and put it in a medium bowl.

- In another larger bowl, mix the leftover fat when you fry the bacon with all the remaining ingredients, either by hand or with a hand blender.

- Put the bowl in the refrigerator for 15 minutes so that the mixture hardens.

- Assemble 24 balls the size of a walnut using two spoons. Bathe in the crumbled bacon and serve.

<u>Advice</u>

- If you prefer, you can use any other type of cheese that has a strong flavor. If you do not eat bacon, you can cover the balls with chopped herbs, grated parmesan cheese or chopped nuts.

- **Keto nougat**

The nougat has always been one of the sweet stars of Christmas.This recipe is crispy and sweet to enjoy at parties without your blood sugar shooting.

<u>Ingredients :</u>

- 225 ml (125 g) macadamia nuts or almonds
- 225 ml (175 g) erythritol
- 2 tbsp Water
- 1 large egg white
- 1 pinch salt

<u>Instructions</u>

- Preheat the oven to 100 ° C (200 ° F).
- Line a pan for bread, about 20 x 15 cm (8x6 inches), with baking paper.

- Put the macadamia nuts in a pan and heat over medium heat until they are golden brown and toasted. Remove from heat and add to bread pan.

- In a small saucepan, combine the erythritol and water. Stir occasionally while heating over medium heat until the mixture is completely liquid.

- While the syrup begins to boil, quickly beat the egg white with the salt until it is white and foamy, almost fluffy.

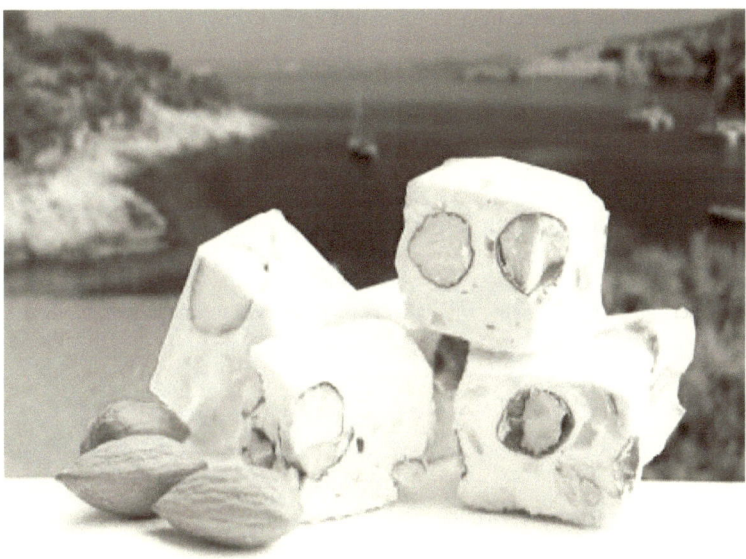

- While you continue beating the eggs, slowly pour the syrup until everything is well mixed.

- Transfer the egg mixture back to the small saucepan and continue stirring with a spatula over low heat until the mixture of egg and syrup is smooth and viscous, about 30 minutes.

- Pour this mixture over the macadamia nuts and level it.

- Place the bread pan in the oven for 2 hours. This is to dry the mixture and make the candy dry.

- Once done, remove from the oven and allow to cool to room temperature before unmolding.

- Cut or break into pieces. Store wrapped in paper at room temperature in a cool, dry place.

- **Chocolate keto cake with peanut butter cream**

 A perfect birthday cake keto ; will delight everyone, even the most sweet tooth. A superesponsive chocolate cake with peanut butter cream glaze .

Ingredients :

- Chocolate cake

- 225 ml (110 g) ground almonds

- 175 ml (125 g) erythritol

- 125 ml (50 g) cocoa powder

- 1½ tbsp (12 g) powdered psyllium husks

- 1 tbsp baking powder

- ¼ tsp. Salt

- 4 eggs

- 225 g (225 ml) cream cheese

- 110 g melted salted butter

- Glazed peanut butter

- 225 g salted butter

- 225 g (225 ml) cream cheese

- 125 ml peanut butter without salt and without sugar

- 60 ml (50 g) erythritol , powder

- 2 tsp vanilla extra

Ornaments

- 10 cherries (optional)

- 125 ml whipping cream

- 1 tbsp (10 g) salted peanuts, chopped

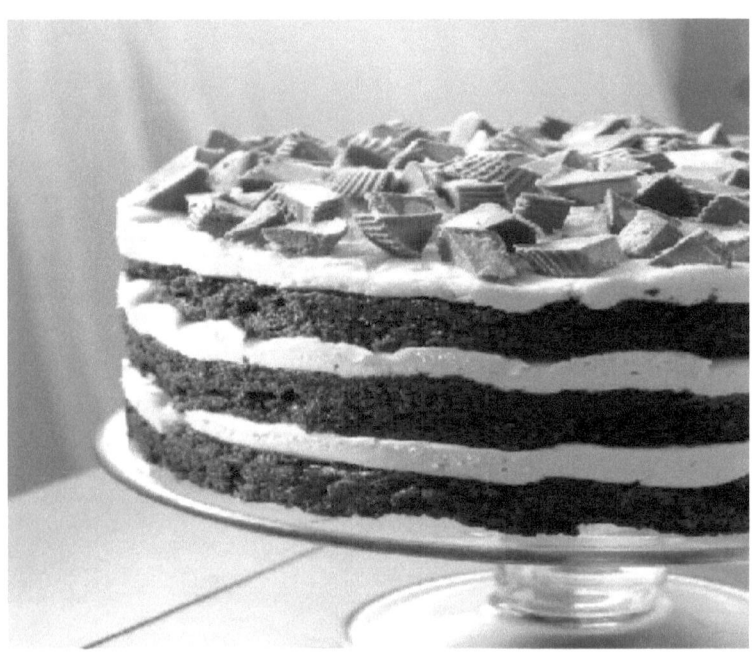

Instructions :

- Place the rack in the center of the oven and preheat to 180 ° C (350 ° F).

- Mix the almond flour, the sweetener, the cocoa powder (filter to remove lumps), the ground psyllium husk powder, the baking powder and the salt in a medium bowl. Beat until well blended. Reserve.

- Pour the eggs in a large bowl. Beat with the electric pastry blender for a couple of minutes until they are spongy. Add the cream cheese and the melted butter. Continue beating until the mixture is smooth and homogeneous.

- Add the flour mixture in the bowl with the eggs and beat a couple of minutes until the dough is smooth.

- Grease two molds for cakes of 18 cm (7 inches), or do it one by one if you only have one mold. Pour half of the dough into each mold and distribute it evenly. Bake for 15-20 minutes or until a toothpick in the center comes out clean.

- Allow to cool for at least 10 minutes in the mold before passing it to a rack to cool. Wrap the layers with plastic wrap and place it in the refrigerator; Allow to cool completely, preferably overnight.

Glazed peanut butter cream

- Mix the butter at room temperature, the cream cheese and the peanut butter in a bowl. Add the sweetener (filter to eliminate lumps) and the vanilla extract. Beat with the electric mixer until smooth.

Assemble the cake

- Place a layer with the flat side up on a plate or on a cake holder. Cover the top with 1/4 of the glaze with a spatula or knife. Place the second layer on top and spread the rest of the glaze on top and on the sides of the cake.

- Beat the cream to beat until it is about to snow and decorate the top with piping bag roses. Put the cherries on top of each piece of cake. Chop the peanuts and sprinkle them on top.

I do not have erythritol powder, what should I do?

- Do not worry, just mix the normal erythritol in a food processor for a couple of minutes until you get a fine powder. You can also use a few drops of liquid stevia as a substitute.

Can I prepare the cake in advance?

- If you make a cake in layers like us, it is better to prepare the layers of the cake one day before serving. Make the frosting the same day you eat it.

Do I have to eat it all at once?

- No, it's not necessary. You can also surprise your neighbors with whatever is left of the cake or cover it and it will stay fresh and fluffy in the refrigerator for at least 2-3 days. Put it in the freezer to keep it fresh up to 3 months. Thaw in the refrigerator overnight.

I do not like peanuts, is there a substitute?

- Do not hesitate to change the peanut butter for any other nut butter you like. Hazelnuts and chocolate are another winning combination. You can also skip it completely and you'll have a tasty vanilla frosting.

Can I do it without almond flour?

- If you can! But the taste and consistency will be very different. 1 cup of almond flour can be substituted for 1/3 of a cup of coconut flour.

- **Keto Brownie Cheesecake**

A creamy keto vanilla cheesecake filling atop a rich brownie crust.

Ingredients :

Brownie Base:

- 1/2 cup butter
- 2 oz unsweetened chocolate chopped
- 1/2 cup almond flour
- 1/4 cup cocoa powder
- pinch salt
- 2 large eggs
- 3/4 cup Swerve Sweetener
- 1/4 tsp vanilla extract
- 1/4 cup walnuts or pecans chopped

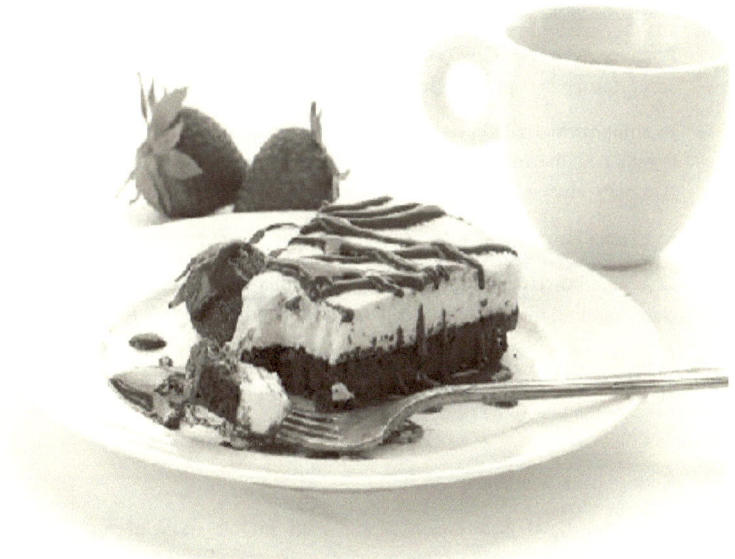

<u>Cheesecake Filling:</u>

- 1 lb cream cheese softened
- 2 large eggs
- 1/2 cup Swerve Sweetener
- 1/4 cup heavy cream
- 1/2 tsp vanilla extract

<u>Instructions :</u>

<u>For the brownie base:</u>

- Preheat oven to 325F and butter a 9-inch springform pan. (if your springform pan is prone to leaking oil, place it on a cookie sheet)
- In a microwave safe bowl or glass measuring cup, melt butter and chocolate together in the microwave in 30 second increments. Whisk until smooth. Alternatively, you can melt them together over low heat in a small saucepan.
- In a small bowl, whisk together almond flour, cocoa powder and salt.
- In a large bowl, beat eggs, Swerve and vanilla until smooth. Beat in almond flour mixture, then butter/chocolate mixture until smooth. Stir in nuts.
- Spread evenly over bottom of prepared pan. Bake 12 to 18 minutes until set around edges but still soft in the center. Let cool 15 to 20 minutes.

<u>For the filling:</u>

- Reduce oven temperature to 300F.
- In a large bowl, beat cream cheese until smooth. Beat in eggs, Swerve, cream and vanilla until well combined.

- Pour filling over crust and place cheesecake on a large cookie sheet. Bake until edges are set and center just barely jiggles, 35 to 45 minutes. Remove from oven and let cool.

- Run a knife around edges to loosen and then remove sides of pan. Cover with plastic wrap and refrigerate at least 3 hours.

- Serve with sugar-free chocolate sauce, if desired.

- **Fudgy Mint Chocolate Cookies**

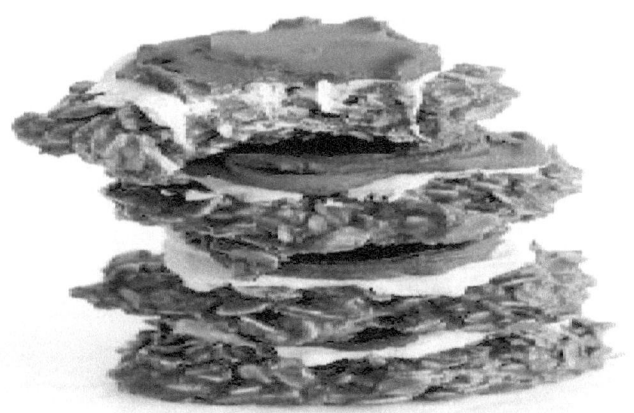

Servings : 24

Ingredients:

- Cookies
- 1/2 cup butter

- 2 cups granulated sugar
- 1/2 cup unsweetened cocoa powder
- 1/2 cup milk
- 1 teaspoon vanilla
- 1/2 teaspoon salt
- 3 1/2 cups oats I use **q**uick
- 2 1/2 cups shredded unsweetened coconut

Frosting :

- 1/2 cup butter room temperature
- 1 1/2 cups icing sugar
- 1 tbsp milk
- 1/2 tsp mint extract
- green food coloring
- Ganache
- 3/4 cup semisweet chocolate chips
- 1 tbsp milk
- 1 tbsp butter

Instructions :

1. Line 2 cookie sheets with wax paper.

2. In a large pot, combine butter, sugar, cocoa and milk. Bring to a boil over medium-high heat, stirring frequently, and boil 1-2 minutes.

3. Stir in vanilla and salt. Add oats and coconut and stir to combine.

4. Drop into 24 spoonfuls onto wax paper. Refrigerate until set.

5. Meanwhile, make the frosting. To a stand mixer (or use a hand mixer), add butter, icing sugar and milk and beat until creamy and blended. Add in mint extract and food coloring. If necessary, add an extra tbsp sugar or milk to achieve the right consistency -- you do not want the icing Runny.

6. Remove cookies from the fridge and spread with frosting. Return to the fridge to let the frosting set.

7. Make the ganache: In a small pot, combine chocolate, milk and butter over very low heat. Cook and stir constantly until chocolate is smooth. Set aside to cool 5-10 minutes. Spread on cooled cookies, and return to the refrigerator to allow chocolate to set.

8. Because they are slightly gooey, you can store them in the fridge or freezer with wax paper between layers so they don't stick together.

- **Keto Blackberry Cheese Bars**

Not only do these blackberry cheesecake bars look amazing but they are delicious as well. Berries are a staple in the keto diet

Ingredients :

For The Crust:
- 1-⅓ cup Almond Flour
- 2 tsp Coconut Flour
- 2 T Butter
- 2 tsp Water
- ⅛ cup Lakanto Golden Sweetener*
- 1 tsp Vanilla
- For the Cream Cheese Layer:
- 8 oz Full Fat Cream Cheese

- 1 tsp Vanilla Extract

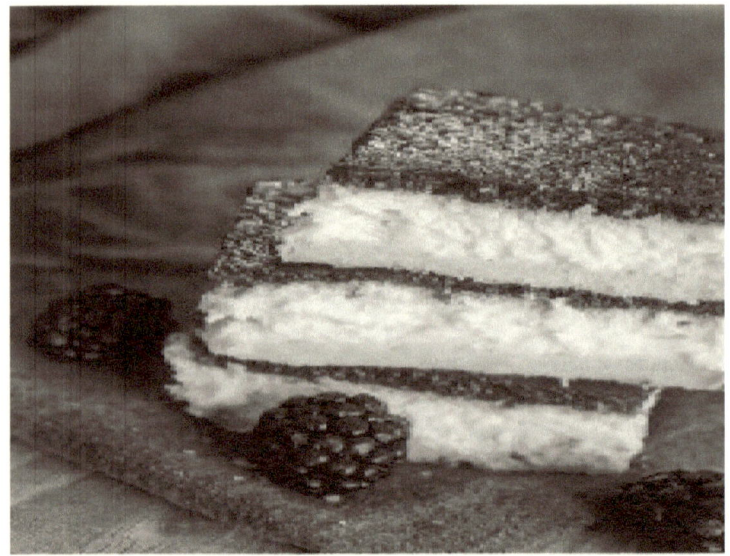

- ½ cup Lakanto Powdered Sweetener*

- 1/2 cup Heavy Whipping Cream

- 1 tsp. Beef Gelatin

For The Blackberry Topping:

- 2.5 cup fresh or frozen Blackberries

- ¾ cup Water

- ⅔ cup Lakanto Classic Sweetener*

- 1 tsp. Lemon Juice

- 1 T Great Lakes or Vital Proteins Gelatin

Instructions :

1. Preheat oven to 350 degrees.

2. Mix all of the pie crust ingredients in a bowl until combined. Press into your 9x9 pan.

3. Bake at 350 for 10-12 minutes until the edges just start to brown. Take out of the oven and let cool completely before mixing up the filling.

4. To make the cream cheese layer, whip 1/2 cup of whipping cream in a large bowl.

5. In a separate bowl, beat the cream cheese, vanilla, Lakanto powdered sweetener, and gelatin.

6. Gently fold the whipped cream in with the cream cheese mixture, until thoroughly combined. Spread evenly in the bottom of the prepared and cooled crust, then place in the refrigerator to cool down while you make the blackberry layer.

7. To make the blueberry layer, bring 1.5 cups of blackberries, the water, Lakanto Classic, lemon juice, and gelatin to a boil in a medium saucepan. Stir well to eliminate clumps.

8. Take off the heat and blend with an immersion blender or in your stand-along blender until smooth and there are no clumps. Stir in the remaining 1 cup of blackberries.

9. Cool the blackberry topping to room temperature, then slowly pour it over the cream cheese layer.

10. Refrigerate 4 hours or overnight to set completely - enjoy!

- **Chocolate Mousse Tart**

Servings : 12

Ingredients :

<u>Crust:</u>

1. 1 1/4 cups almond flour
2. 1/4 cup cocoa powder
3. 1/4 cup powdered Swerve Sweetener
4. 5 tbsp butter melted

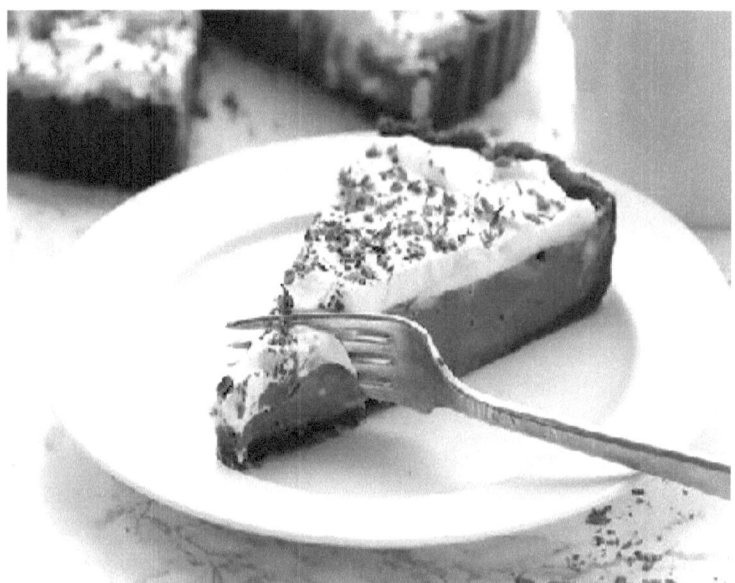

<u>Chocolate Mousse Filling:</u>

1. 3/4 cup whipping cream
2. 3/4 cup unsweetened nut milk
3. 1/4 cup butter

4. 3 ounces good quality unsweetened dark chocolate chopped (do not use sweetened chocolate here, as your mousse may not set properly)

5. 3 tbsp cocoa powder

6. 6 tbsp powdered Swerve Sweetener

7. 1/2 tsp espresso powder optional, boosts chocolate flavour

8. 3 large eggs

Topping:

- 1 cup whipping cream

- 2 tbsp powdered Swerve Sweetener

- 1/4 tsp vanilla extract

- 1/2 ounce dark sugar-free chocolate

Instructions :

Crust:

1. Lightly grease a 9-inch tart pan with a removable bottom.

2. In a medium bowl, whisk together the almond flour, cocoa powder, and sweetener. Add melted butter and stir until the mixture clumps together.

3. Press firmly and evenly into bottom and up sides of prepared tart pan. Refrigerate until filling is ready.

4. Chocolate Mousse:

5. In a small pan, combine cream, almond or cashew milk, and butter. Bring to a full boil and then remove from heat.

6. In a blender, combine unsweetened chocolate, cocoa powder, sweetener, and espresso powder. Pour in scalded cream mixture and blend until smooth.

7. Add eggs and blend again until smooth (*if you are concerned about the eggs, use pasteurized shell eggs such as Safest Choice). Pour into chilled

crust and chill until firm, at least 1 hour. Gently press the tart pan from the bottom to remove the sides and place on a serving platter.

<u>Topping:</u>

1. Beat whipping cream with sweetener and vanilla until it holds stiff peaks. Spread over mousse to the edges of the tart.

2. Using a cheese grater, shave the dark chocolate over the whipping cream. Let set a bit in the refrigerator before serving.

- **Low Carb Cheesecake**

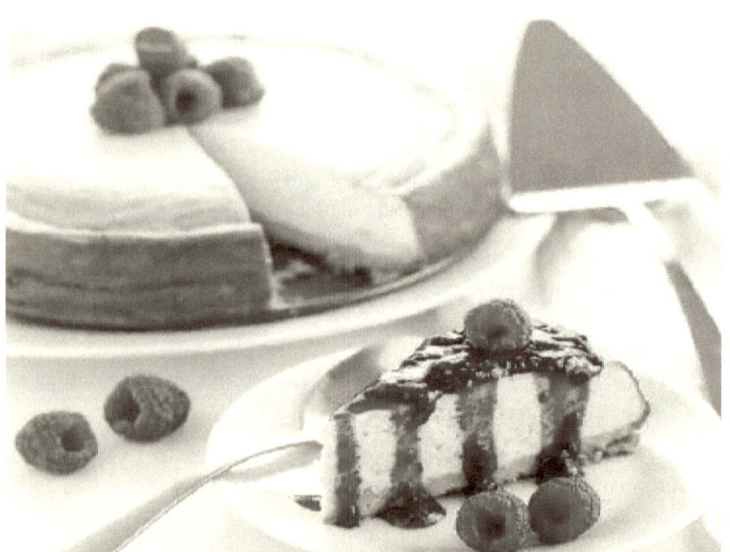

Serving: 16 Slice

Ingredients :

- Almond Flour Cheesecake Crust
- 2 cups Blanched almond flour
- 1/3 cup Butter (measured solid, then melted)
- 3 tbsp Erythritol (granular or powdered works fine)
- 1 tsp Vanilla extract
- Keto Cheesecake Filling
- 32 oz Cream cheese (softened)
- 1 1/4 cup Powdered erythritol (erythritol must be powdered; can also use powdered monk fruit sweetener)
- 3 large Egg
- 1 tbsp Lemon juice
- 1 tsp Vanilla extract

Instructions :

1. Preheat the oven to 350 degrees F (177 degrees C). Grease a 9 in (23 cm) springform pan (or you can line the bottom with parchment paper).

2. To make the almond flour cheesecake crust, stir the almond flour, melted butter, erythritol, and vanilla extract in a medium bowl, until well combined. The dough will be slightly crumbly. Press the dough into the bottom of the prepared pan. Bake for about 10-12 minutes, until barely golden. Let cool at least 10 minutes.

3. Meanwhile, beat the cream cheese and powdered sweetener together at low to medium speed until fluffy. Beat in the eggs, one at a time. Finally, beat in the lemon juice and vanilla extract. (Keep the mixer at low to medium the

whole time; too high speed will introduce too many air bubbles, which we don't want.)

4. Pour the filling into the pan over the crust. Smooth the top with a spatula (use a pastry spatula for a smoother top if you have one).

5. Bake for about 45-55 minutes, until the center is almost set, but still jiggly.

6. Remove the cheesecake from the oven. If the edges are stuck to the pan, run a knife around the edge (don't remove the springform edge yet). Cool in the pan on the counter to room temperature, then refrigerate for at least 4 hours (preferably overnight), until completely set. (Do not try to remove the cake from the pan before chilling.)

7. Serve with fresh raspberry sauce if desired.*

Note

To make optional raspberry sauce, simmer 1 cup fresh raspberries with 2 tablespoons water and sweetener to taste, for 5-10 minutes, breaking the berries with a spatula. Add additional water to thin out to your liking.

* **Keto Pecan Pie Cheesecake**

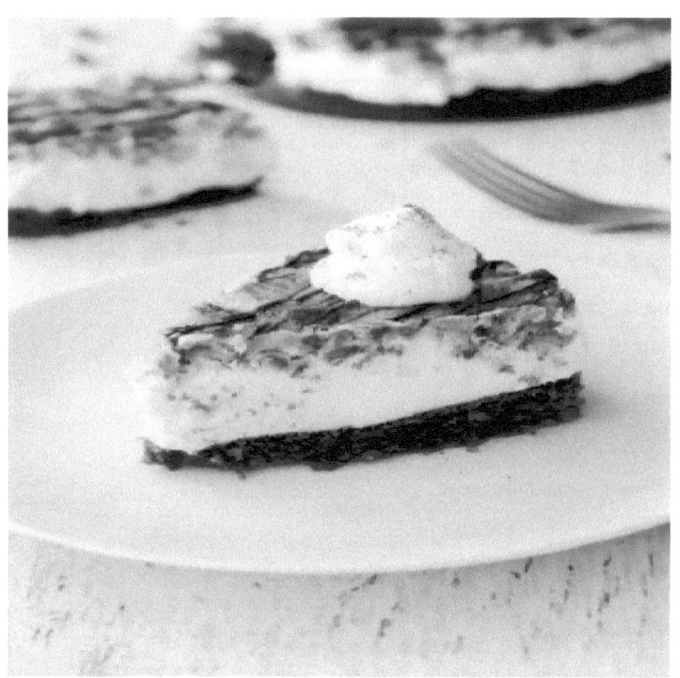

Serving : 12 Slice

Ingredients:

Crust :

- 1 1/3 cup Pecans
- 1 tbsp Cacao Powder
- 2 tbsp Swerve Confectioner Sweetener , or preferred sweetener
- 1 tsp Vanilla Extract
- 3 tbsp cold butter

Cheesecake Layer :

- 16 oz Cream Cheese
- 1 cup Swerve Confectioner Sweetener, or preferred sweetener
- 2/3 cup Heavy Whipping Cream
- 2 tsp Vanilla Extract
- Caramel Layer
- 5 tbsp Butter; divided
- 1/2 cup Swerve Confectioner Sweetener , or choice of sweetener
- 2 tbsp Heavy Whipping Cream
- 1/2 tsp Vanilla Extract
- 1 1/2 cup Chopped Pecans

Instructions :

crust

1. Preheat Oven to 350.
2. Place all crust ingredients in food processor and pulse until soft dough forms. Press dough into greased 7 inch springform pan. Bake for 12-15 minutes. Set aside, let cool.
3. cheesecake layer
4. In large mixing bowl, place softened cream cheese and beat for 3 minutes until completely smooth. Add swerve, or preferred sweetener and beat additional 3 minutes.
5. Add heavy whipping cream and vanilla. Whip for 5-7 minutes or until mixture is completely smooth.
6. Pour mixture onto cooled (or mostly cooled) crust and spread evenly. Place in freezer while you prepare final layer.

7. caramel pecan layer

8. In skillet or saucepan over medium-low heat add 4 tbsp butter. Once butter is almost completely melted add swerve, or choice of sweetener. Stir frequently with rubber spatula and watch closely as it turns golden brown.

9. Once it is light or golden brown, add heavy cream and pecans. Continue gentle stirring frequently until dark golden brown. Turn off heat and add final tablespoon of butter. Let mixture cool for 10 minutes.

10. Mixture should still very hot but cooled from the near boiling point. Remove cheesecake from freezer and pour caramel pecan mixture over top, using rubber spatula to even layer. Try to make sure all pecan pieces are flat and level with caramel for best results. You may need to press them down gently or gently move pan back and forth to level.

11. Place in fridge overnight to completely cool. If mixture is not completely cool when cut into, the top layer will not stay together.

12. Place in freezer for 2-3 hours before you're going to eat it. Freezing it will firm up the cheesecake layer and allow you to slice through the top layer without it cracking.

Notes

You may use the sweetener of your choice. You may use unsweetened cocoa powder in place of cacao, you may need to add additional sweetener,to taste. Make sure top pecan layer is completely cooled before cutting or it may fall apart. The cheesecake layer is a no-bake cheesecake. The only thing cooked in the oven in this recipe is the crust.

- **No Bake Keto Coconut Cookies**

Serving : 20 Cookies

Ingredients :

- 3 cups shredded unsweetened coconut flakes I used finely shredded

- 1 cup coconut oil, melted
- 1/2 cup monk fruit sweetened maple syrup Can substitute for any liquid sweetener of choice- See notes

Instructions :

1. Line a large plate or baking tray with parchment paper and set aside.

2. In a large mixing bowl, combine all your ingredients and mix very well. Lightly wet your hands then form small balls with the batter, placing them 1-2 inches apart on the lined baking tray.

3. Using a fork, press down onto each cookie. Refrigerate until firm.

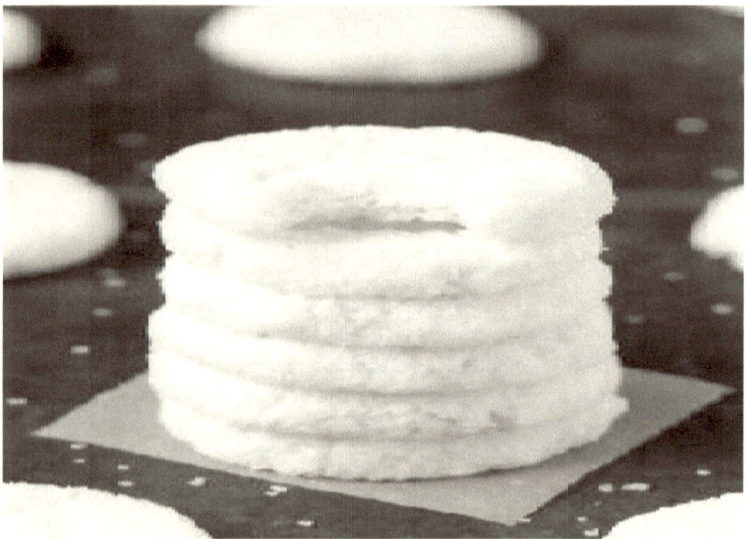

Notes : Depending on the texture you are after, you could reduce the amount of sticky sweetener to 1/4 cup. 3-Ingredient Paleo Vegan No Bake Coconut Cookies can be kept at room temperature (covered) for up to 7 days. They can be refrigerated for up to a month and frozen for up to 2 months.

- **Keto Chocolate Coffee Fat Bombs**

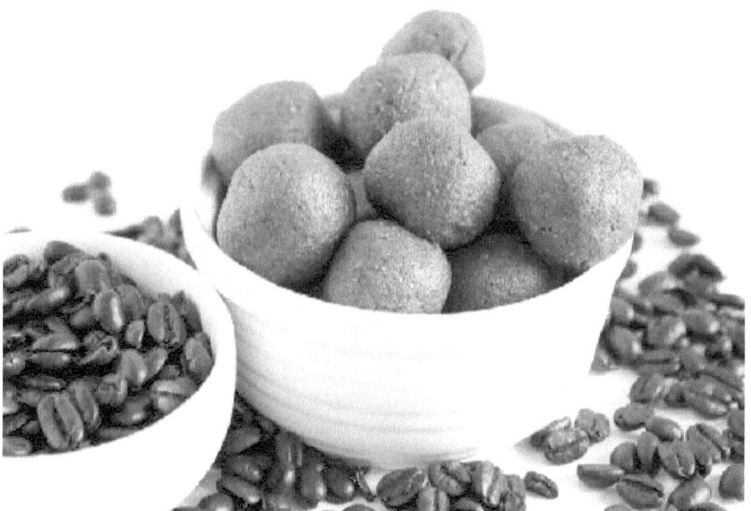

These keto chocolate coffee fat bombs are super delicious.Each contains 9g fat,1g net carbs and they are caffeinated.If you love the taste of coffee,you have to try out this.This combination is everything.Coffee + chocolate you get delicious keto fat bombs.

Ingredients :

- 2 1/2 c pecans
- 2 tbsp instant coffee granules
- 2 1/2 tbsp Dutch-process cocoa powder

- 3/4 tsp stevia
- 1 tbsp coconut oil

Instructions :

1. Into food processor bowl, add all ingredients except coconut oil. Pulse ten times to incorporate everything, then add coconut oil.

2. Pulse mixture for 1 1/2 to 2 minutes, scraping down the sides every 30 seconds, until the mixture starts to have the ability to stick together. Be careful not to process it to the point of being nut butter!

3. Roll into 20 fat bombs (approximately 1 tbsp of the mixture per fat bomb). To form them, you'll need to squish together the mixture a few times in your hands to get it to stick together, then roll it into a ball shape. (Note: If your mixture is too sticky and doesn't hold together well enough, quickly pulse in 1-2 tbsp almond flour.)

4. Optionally, roll the fat bombs in a coating (see recipe notes for ideas).

5. Place fat bombs on a plate and refrigerate for at least 45 minutes. These are soft fat bombs, so they won't really firm up; chilling them just gives time for the flavors to incorporate. Store them in the fridge.

- **Easy chocolate keto fat bombs**

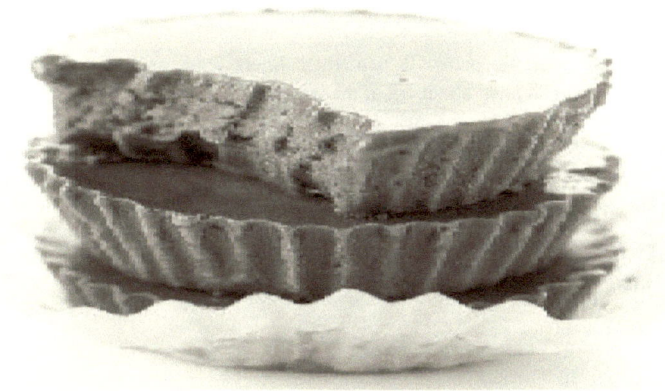

Serving: 20

Ingredients :

- 2 cup Macadamia nuts (dry roasted, salted)
- 2 tbsp Coconut oil (measured solid, then melted)
- 2 tbsp MCT oil (or more coconut oil for firmer fat bombs)
- 1 tsp Vanilla extract (optional)
- 1/3 cup Powdered monk fruit sweetener
- 1/4 cup Cocoa powder

Instructions :

1. Pulse/puree macadamia nuts into a food processor or high power blender, until mostly broken down into small pieces. Add MCT oil, melted coconut oil, and vanilla. Continue to puree until nut butter forms. (Try to get it

smooth, but if you can't get rid of some stray pieces, that's okay!) Scrape down the sides as necessary.

2. Add the cocoa powder and sweetener gradually, a couple tablespoons at a time. Puree after each addition, until smooth.

3. Line a mini muffin pan with parchment liners. Pour or spoon the batter evenly into each liner, about 1/3 of the way full.

4. Freeze for at least 30 minutes, until solid.

* **Keto Blueberry Cream Pie Fat Bombs**

Ingredients:

- 4 oz soft goat cheese
- 1/2 cup fresh blueberries
- 1 cup almond flour
- 1 tsp vanilla extract
- 1/2 cup pecans
- 1/2 tsp stevia
- 1/4 cup unsweetened shredded coconut to roll fat bombs .

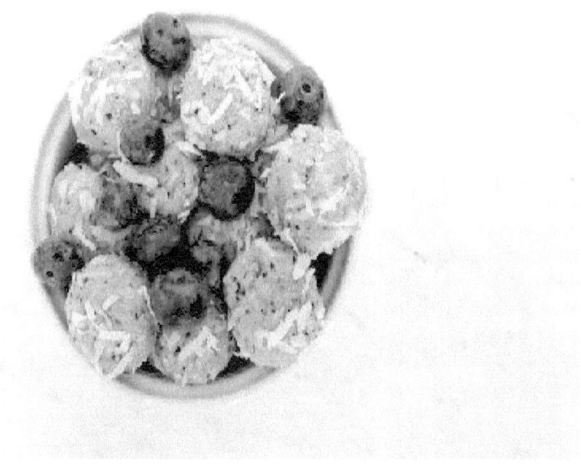

Instructions :

1. Process all ingredients in a food processor until well combined.

2. Roll into 30 small fat bombs.

3. Pour coconut flakes into a small bowl and lightly roll each fat bomb in the shredded coconut.

Notes

Store in fridge until ready to serve.

Keto Soup Recipes

- **Low carb instant pot cauliflower soup**

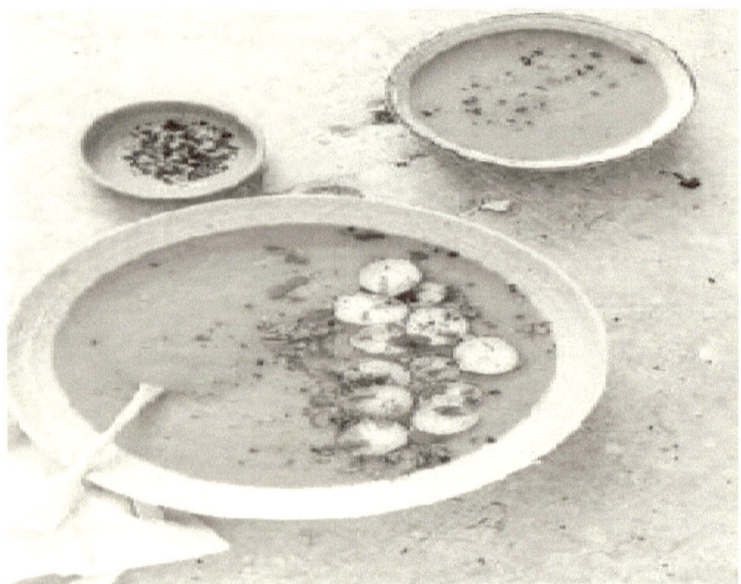

Are you looking for a low carb soup recipe for weeknight dinners? Try this one, you won't be disappointed. It's creamy, smooth, comforting and easy to make.

Ingredients

- 1 tbsp olive oil
- 2 onion peeled and finely chopped

- 1 pepper, deseeded and finely chopped

- 1 bay leaf optional

- 1 tsp garlic puree

- 1.5 tsp smoked paprika

- 1.5 tsp ground cumin

- Chilli to taste

- 1 head of a large cauliflower approx 675 g /1.5lb cut into florets

- 750 ml 3 cups vegetable stock

- Salt

Instructions:

Instant Pot Cauliflower Soup

1. Switch the Instant Pot on to the saute setting and add the oil to the Instant Pot Insert and saute the onions, peppers and bay leaf if using for 4-5 mins until the onion is soft.

2. Switch off the heat and stir in the garlic, paprika, cumin and chilli.

3. Mix in the cauliflower florets, vegetable stock and salt.

4. Cover your Instant Pot, set the vent to 'sealing,' select the manual or pressure cook button (dependent upon IP model), select high pressure and set the timer to 7 mins.

5. When done allow the pot to NPR for 15 mins before releasing the rest of the steam using quick release.

6. Let cool for a few mins, before removing bay leaf and pureeing with an immersion blender.

7. Garnish and serve.

Stove Top Cauliflower Soup

1. Saute the onions, peppers and bay leaf in a pot over medium heat until onions are soft.

2. Stir in the garlic, paprika, cumin and chilli followed by the cauliflower florets, vegetable stock and salt.

3. Cover and simmer for 20 mins until the cauliflower is cooked through.

4. Let cool for a few mins, before removing bay leaf and pureeing with an immersion blender.

- **Keto Creamy Spinach Artichoke Soup**

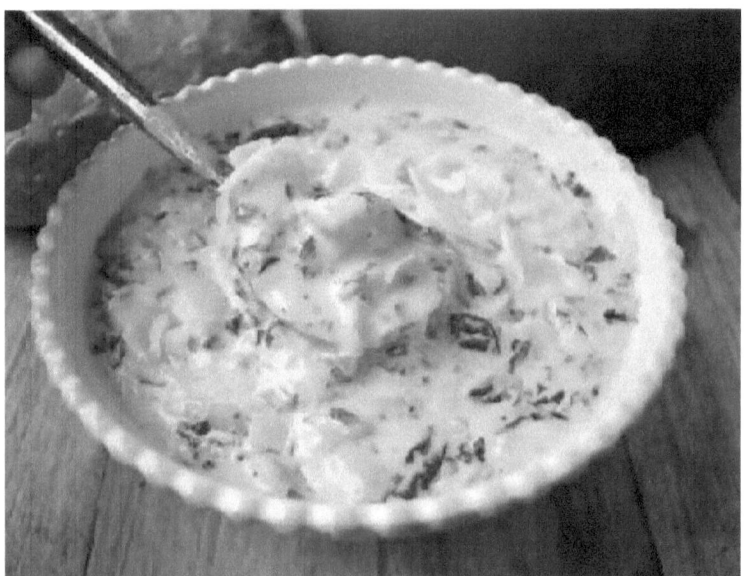

This is one of the low carb keto soup recipes that you can eat all day,everyday.it's easy to make, super healthy, rich, creamy and it's made with spinach, artichoke, chicken broth, cream cheese and garlic.Perfect for the cold winter days. It will keep you full and warm.

Servings : 6

Ingredients :

- 2 Tablespoons Butter
- 1 Onion chopped
- 4 Garlic Cloves minced (or 3/4 teaspoon Garlic Powder)
- 1 - 9- ounce pkg. Frozen Chopped Spinach may use 1/2 of pkg. if you so desire
- 1 teaspoon Salt
- 1 teaspoon Pepper
- 3 Tablespoons Flour may delete if you want gluten-free or keto-friendly soup
- 4 cups Chicken Broth
- 1 - 14 ounce can Artichoke Hearts drained and roughly chopped
- 1 1/2 cups Heavy Cream depending on how creamy you want the soup
- 1 - 8- ounce pkg. Cream Cheese
- 1 cup Parmesan Cheese plus additional 1/2 cup for garnish

Instructions :

1. In a large pot, melt butter over medium-high heat. Add onion and saute for 5 minutes. Add garlic and saute for 1 minute longer.

2. Stir in frozen spinach. Stir often and break apart using a wooden spoon. Cook for 5-7 minutes or until spinach is warmed throughout. Sprinkle with salt and pepper. Stir in flour, stirring well to avoid any lumps.

3. Pour in chicken broth and artichoke hearts. Heat for 5-10 minutes.

4. Turn heat to LOW. Add heavy cream. Stir together. Add cream cheese and let melt slowly. You want it to be at a low heat to prevent curdling.

5. Stir in parmesan cheese.

6. Season according to taste. Sprinkle with parmesan cheese shavings.

Note: If you want to make this Creamy Spinach Artichoke Soup keto-friendly, you can remove the flour from the recipe. The flour serves as a thickening agent

- **Low Carb Chili Recipe**

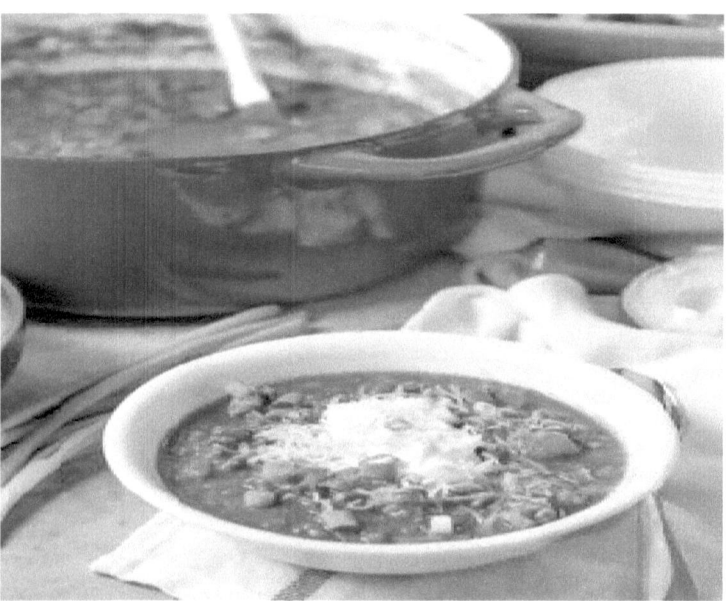

ServingS : 4

Ingredients:

- 1 pound ground beef
- 2 cloves of garlic, minced (or 1/2 tsp garlic powder)
- 1 large bell pepper (your favorite color)
- about 1 cup onion, diced (use more if you like sauteed onion)
- 2 tsp chili powder
- 1 tsp cumin
- 1/4 tsp pepper
- 1 tsp salt (You could cheat and just use 2 tbs of a chili spice mix in place of the 4 spices above.)
- 1 tsp Worcestershire
- 1/2 tsp celery salt
- 4 oz can diced green chiles
- 1 cup of tomato sauce
- 1 cup beef broth
- 1 tbs tomato paste

Instructions :

1. Combine the ground beef, onions, bell peppers and garlic in large frying pan and sauté until ground beef is browned. Drain fat.

2. Add spices, Worcestershire, diced green chiles, tomato sauce, tomato paste and broth to the pan. stir to combine and simmer for 30 minutes to an hour.

3. Give chili a taste, add additional cumin, chili powder and additional cayenne if desired.

- **Keto Roasted Red Pepper Soup**

Servings : 2

Ingredients :

- 0.42 lb sweet peppers
- 0.17 lb chopped cauliflower
- 0.33 cups chicken broth
- 0.33 cups heavy cream
- 0.25 tsp salt
- 0.17 tsp sugar-free sweetener optional
- 0.33 scoops Vital Proteins Chicken Bone Broth Collagen

Instructions :

1. Put the sweet peppers on a large baking sheet. Roast at 400 degrees for 30 minutes or until softened and slightly browned.

2. Meanwhile, add the cauliflower and broth to a large stock pot. Simmer over medium until the peppers are done. Stir in the bone broth collagen.

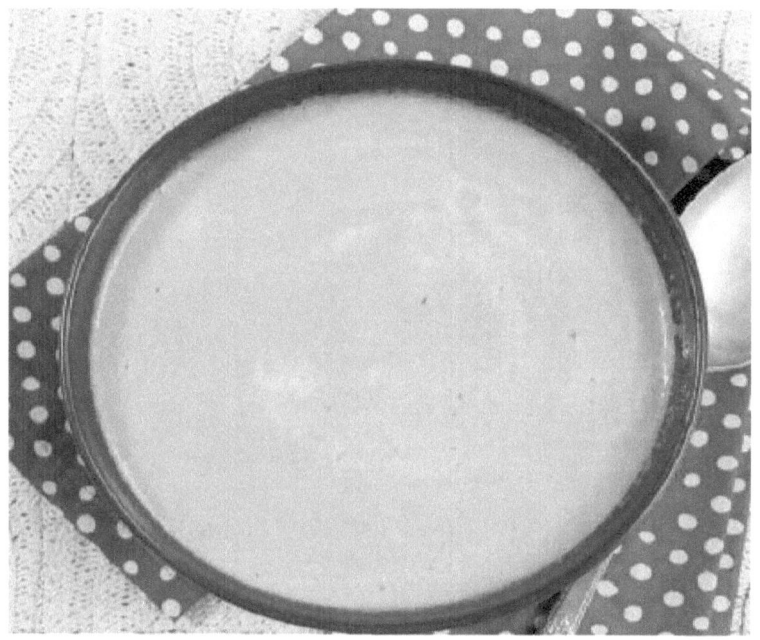

3. Add the peppers, cauliflower, half the broth, and the remaining ingredients to a blender. Process until smooth. Add back to the pot and heat until hot.

- **Keto Vegan Cream Of Tomato Soup**

Servings : 4

Ingredients :

- 4 (375 grams) roma tomatoes
- ½ cup (85 grams) sun dried tomatoes
- ½ cup raw macadamia nuts
- 1 teaspoon sea salt

- ¼ cup (20 grams) fresh basil
- ½ teaspoon white pepper
- ¼ teaspoon black pepper
- 1 clove garlic
- 4 cups hot water

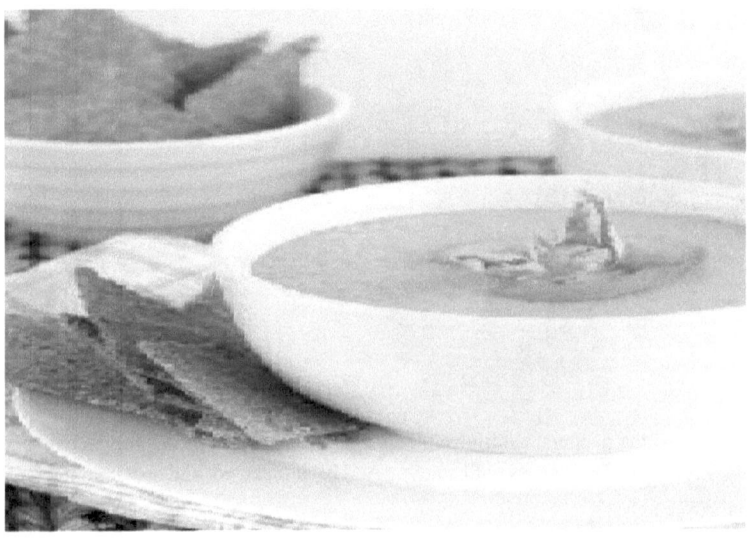

Instructions :

1. Add all ingredients to the jug of your high-powered blender and blend, on high, for 5 minutes until heated through.

2. Serve with a side of homemade sweet potato tortilla chips, if desired.

- **Unstuffed Cabbage Roll Soup**

Ingredients :

- 28 ounce can diced tomatoes
- 1 pound 90% lean ground beef
- 1 pound chopped green cabbage (about 5 cups)
- 5 cups beef stock
- 1 cup riced cauliflower
- 1/2 cup diced onions
- 1/2 cup diced carrots

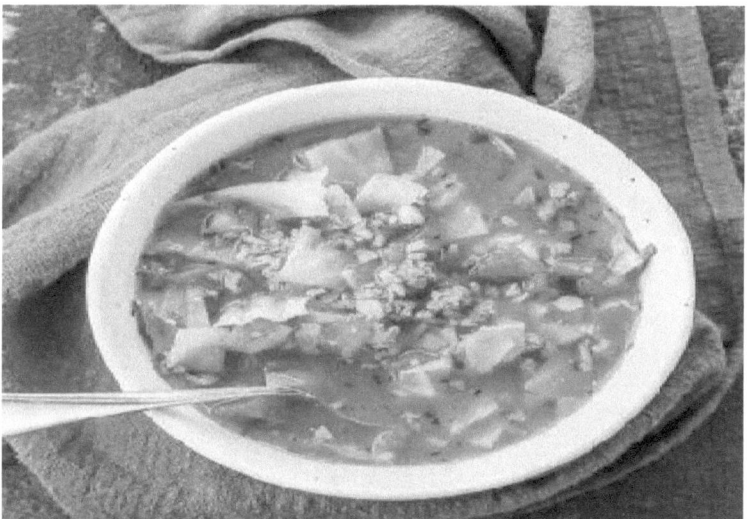

- 1 tablespoon olive oil
- 1 1/2 teaspoons salt
- 1 teaspoon dried oregano

- 1 teaspoon dried thyme
- 2 tablespoons fresh chopped parsley

Instructions :

1. Heat a 6 quart pot or dutch oven over medium to medium-high heat. Add olive oil and ground beef, cooking for a few minutes until browned, breaking it apart as it cooks.

2. Add onions and carrots. Cook for a few minutes to soften, stirring frequently.

3. Add tomatoes (including the liquid in the can), cabbage, beef stock, cauliflower, oregano, thyme, and salt. Stir everything together.

4. Increase heat to bring to a simmer. Cover with a lid and decrease heat to maintain a simmer. Simmer for about 30 minutes or until cabbage is tender.

5. Uncover and stir. Top with parsley and serve while hot.

- **Easy Keto Lobster Bisque Soup Recipe**

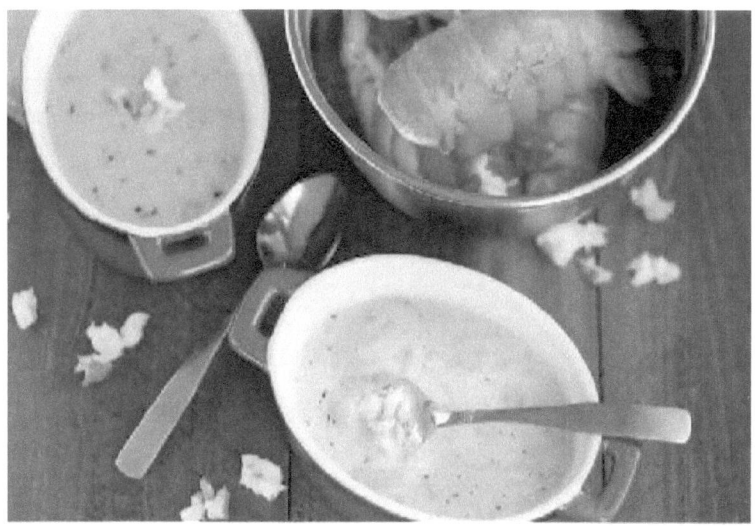

Servings : 2

Ingredients :

- 1.33 lobster tails frozen in shells (or fresh)
- 0.67 tablespoons olive oil extra virgin
- 0.17 cup onion chopped
- 0.5 teaspoons garlic minced
- 0.33 cup dry white wine
- 0.67 teaspoons Worcestershire sauce
- 0.33 teaspoon celery salt
- 0.33 teaspoon dried thyme
- 0.17 teaspoon paprika

- 0.17 teaspoon ground cayenne pepper
- 0.08 teaspoon ground black pepper
- 0.33 tablespoon tomato paste increase to 2 tablespoons for more tomato flavor
- 0.67 cups lobster stock
- 0.67 cups heavy cream
- 1.33 tablespoons butter

Instructions :

1. Boil lobster tails for 6-8 minutes or until shells are bright red. Remove tails to cool and reserve water to use as lobster stock.

2. Remove meat from shells then return the shell to water and boil for another 10 minutes. Using fine mesh strainer, strain lobster stock and reserve 2 cups.

3. Chop lobster meat into bite sized pieces. Set aside.

4. Add olive oil to medium sized sauce pan and heat over medium high heat. Saute onion and garlic and cook for about 5 minutes.

5. Slowly add the wine, then stir in the Worcestershire, celery salt, thyme, paprika, cayenne pepper, and black pepper.

6. Stir in the tomato paste and reserved lobster stock. Simmer about 10 minutes.

7. Puree mixture in blender or use a stick blender in the pot until smooth.

8. Return mixture to pot, if needed, and add in the heavy cream and butter. Add additional salt if needed.

9. Add lobster meat and continue to simmer for another 5-10 minutes.

Notes : The soup can be thickened with glucomannan powder, xanthan gum, and or guar gum. Traditional lobster bisque soups were also thickened with ground lobster shells. It's best to use a stick blender right in the pot to puree the soup mixture.

- **Creamy Ham And Cheese Cauliflower Soup**

Ingredients :

- 2 Tbsp vegetable oil for cooking

- 1 small yellow onion

- .75 lb ham

- 2 garlic cloves pressed

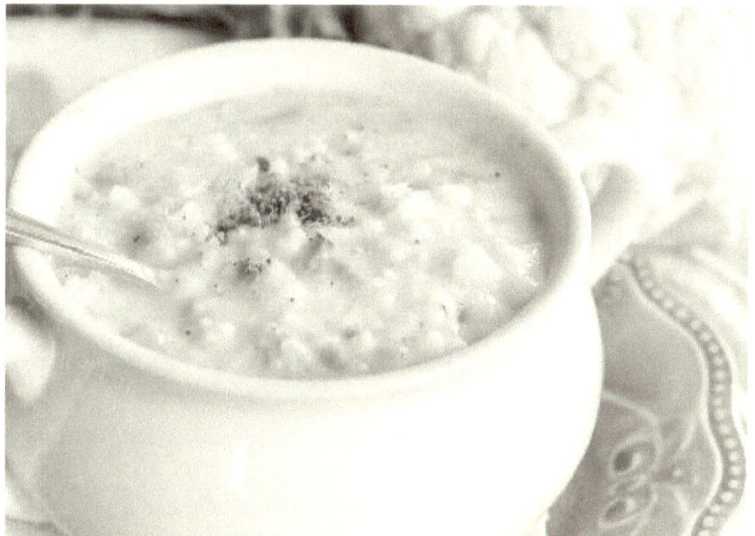

- 2 lb head of cauliflower

- 1 1/2 Tbsp flour

- 1 tsp dry sage

- Salt
- Fresh cracked black pepper
- 3-4 cups chicken stock
- 1 bay leaf
- 1/4 cup heavy whipping cream
- 4 oz sharp white cheddar cheese grated

Instructions :

1. Dice onion and set aside. Dice ham into small pieces and set aside. Cut cauliflower florets off, discard the stem, and chop florets onto small pieces. Set it aside as well.

2. Preheat a medium pot over medium heat with some oil. Add diced onion and saute until transparent. Add ham and cook for a few minutes. Add pressed garlic, mix, and cook until fragrant.

3. Add prepared cauliflower, mix well and cook for a few minutes.

4. Sprinkle flour over veggies and ham and mix well.

5. Pour in chicken stock, while slowly stirring. Enough chicken stock to just covers the cauliflower mixture.

6. Add bay leaf, salt, pepper, and sage. Stir and cover with a lid, leaving a crack for steam to escape. Cook for 20-25 minutes.

7. Stir in heavy whipping cream and grated white cheddar cheese. Cook for a few more minutes and serve.

Keto Chicken Recipes

- **Herbed Chicken And Mushrooms**

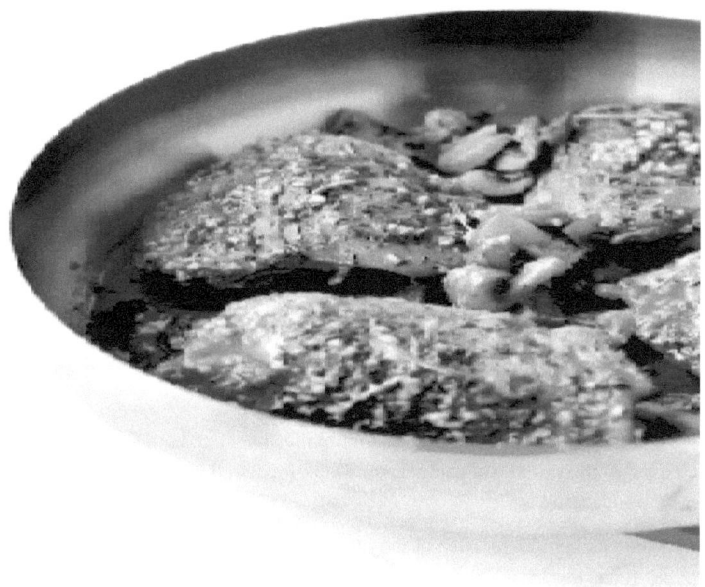

Servings : 4

Ingredients :

- 8 skin-on chicken thighs

- 2 teaspoons sea salt
- 1/2 teaspoon black pepper
- 1 tablespoon plus 1 teaspoon dried oregano
- 1 tablespoon plus 1 teaspoon dried thyme
- 1 tablespoon plus 1 teaspoon dried rosemary
- 2 tablespoons olive oil
- 8 ounces cremini mushrooms, quartered
- 2 cloves garlic, minced
- 1 cup chicken stock
- 2 tablespoons Dijon mustard
- Torn fresh parsley, optional as garnish

Instructions :

1. Preheat the oven to 400°F.
2. Season the chicken thighs on both sides with salt, pepper, 2 teaspoons of the oregano, 2 teaspoons of the dried thyme, and 2 teaspoons of the dried rosemary.
3. Heat the olive oil in a large cast iron skillet over medium heat. Add the chicken to the skillet, skin side down. Cook for 5 to 6 minutes until the skin is nice and crispy.
4. Flip the chicken thighs over to the other side and transfer the skillet to the oven. Bake for 15 to 20 minutes, until the chicken is cooked all the way through.
5. Transfer the skillet back to the stovetop. Remove the chicken from the pan, set aside, and cover to keep warm.
6. To the same skillet, add the mushrooms and cook over medium heat for 5 minutes, until they have releases their liquid and are tender.

7. Add the garlic, chicken stock, Dijon mustard, and the remaining seasonings and cook for an additional 3 minutes.

8. Plate the chicken and pour the sauce over top. Garnish with fresh parsley, if desired.

- **Keto Butter Chicken**

Ingredients:

- 1.5 lbs chicken breast
- 2 tablespoons garam masala
- 3 teaspoons fresh ginger, grated
- 3 teaspoons minced garlic
- 4 oz plain yogurt

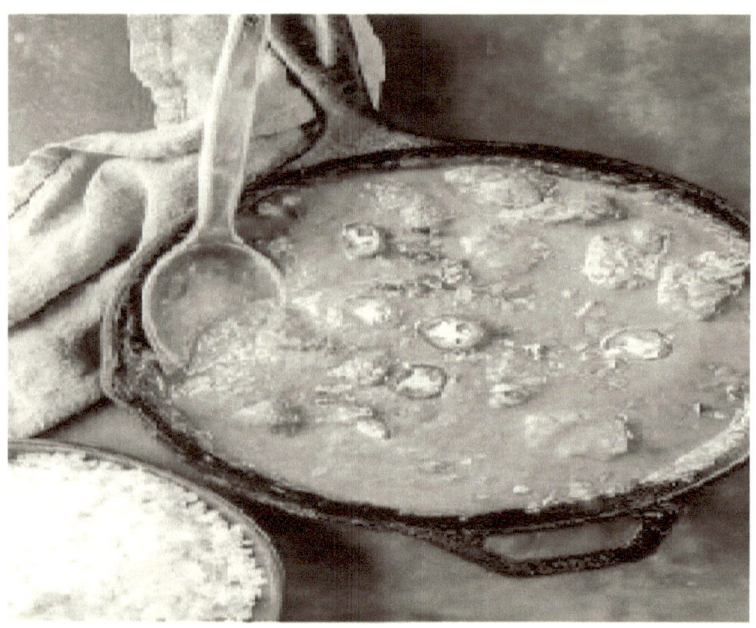

<u>Sauce:</u>

- 2 tablespoons ghee or butter
- 1 onion
- 2 teaspoons fresh ginger, grated
- 2 teaspoons minced garlic
- 14.5 oz crushed tomatoes
- 1 tablespoon ground coriander
- ½ tablespoon garam masala
- 2 teaspoons cumin

- 1 teaspoon chili powder

- ½ cup heavy cream

- Salt, to taste

Optional:

- cilantro

- cauliflower rice

Instructions :

1. Cut chicken into 2 inch pieces and place in a large bowl with 2 tablespoons garam masala, 1 teaspoon grated ginger, and 1 teaspoon minced garlic. Add in the yogurt, stir to combine. Chill at least 30 minutes.

2. For the sauce, place the onion, ginger, garlic, crushed tomatoes and spices in a blender, and blend until smooth. Set aside.

3. Heat 1 tablespoon of oil in a large skillet over medium high heat. Place the chicken in the skillet, browning 3 to 4 minutes per side. Once browned pour in the sauce cook 5 to 6 minutes longer.

4. Stir in the heavy cream and ghee, continue to cook another minute. Taste for salt and add additional if needed. Top with cilantro and serve with cauliflower rice if desired.

- **Keto Chicken Florentine In A Skillet**

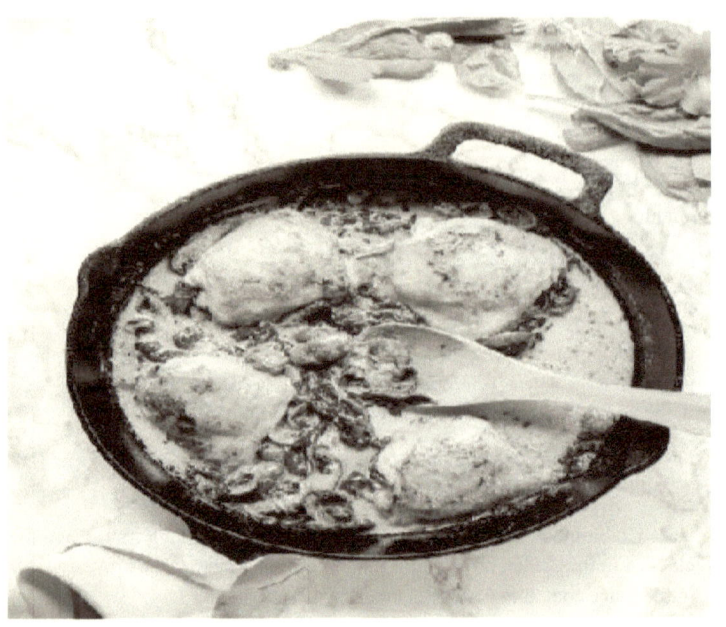

Ingredients :

- 4 bone-in, skin-on chicken thighs
- 2 T avocado oil
- 3/4 C chicken stock or bone broth
- 1 C organic heavy whipping cream
- 1/2 tsp pink Himalayan sea salt
- 1/4 tsp black pepper
- 1/2 tsp Italian seasoning
- 1/2 tsp onion powder

- 1/2 tsp garlic powder
- 8 oz baby bella mushrooms, sliced
- 3/4 C shredded parmesan cheese
- 3 C spinach

Instructions :

1. In a cast iron skillet (or stainless steel pan), heat the avocado oil over medium high heat.

2. Add chicken thighs and cook for 6-8 minutes each side. Skin should turn golden brown and chicken should be almost fully cooked.

3. Remove chicken from skillet and place on a plate.

4. Add chicken stock, heavy whipping cream and spices to skillet.

5. Stir occasionally and reduce heat to low once mixture starts to simmer.

6. Add mushrooms and cook until softened.

7. Add spinach and Parmesan cheese. Stir until cheese is melted.

8. Add chicken back into skillet and cook for an additional 3-5 minutes, stirring occasionally until chicken is fully cooked. Make sure internal temperature of chicken reaches 165 F.

- **Keto Chicken Enchiladas**

Servings : 3

Ingredients:

- 1 lb chicken, boiled and shredded
- 1 medium onion, sliced (165g)
- 1 4 oz can green chilies

- 3 zucchinis (285g) cut into strips
- 1 tbsp oil
- 8 oz shredded jack cheese
- 1 cup enchilada sauce

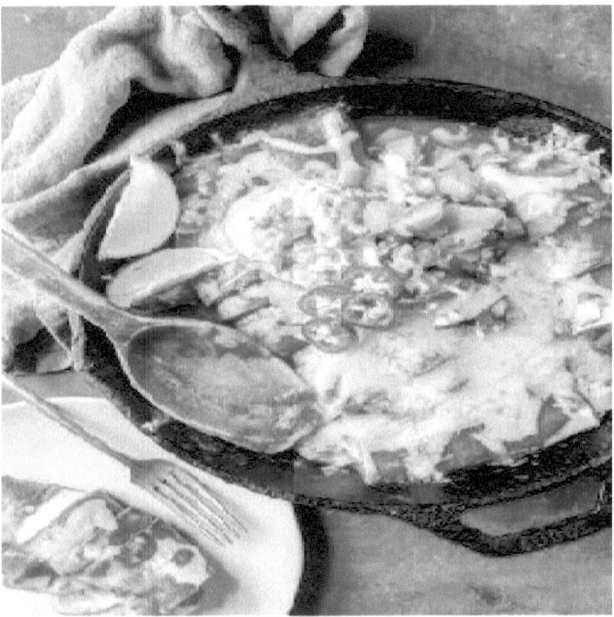

optional toppings:

- sour cream
- guacamole
- pico de gallo

- jalapeno
- cilantro

Instructions:

1. Preheat broiler to high heat.

2. Heat oil in a medium skillet over medium heat, saute onion 3 to 4 minutes until soft. Stir in green chilis and shredded chicken, remove from heat and stir in half of the cheese.

3. Cut the zucchini into long flat sheets using a mandoline or vegetable peeler. Layer 4 pieces slightly overlapping and place 1/4 cup of filling at the end of the strips. Carefully roll up and place in a cast iron skillet.

4. Top the zucchini enchiladas with the enchilada sauce and the remaining cheese. Broil in over for 5-7 minutes until cheese is bubbly. Serve with desired toppings.

- **Chicken And Avocado Tacos**

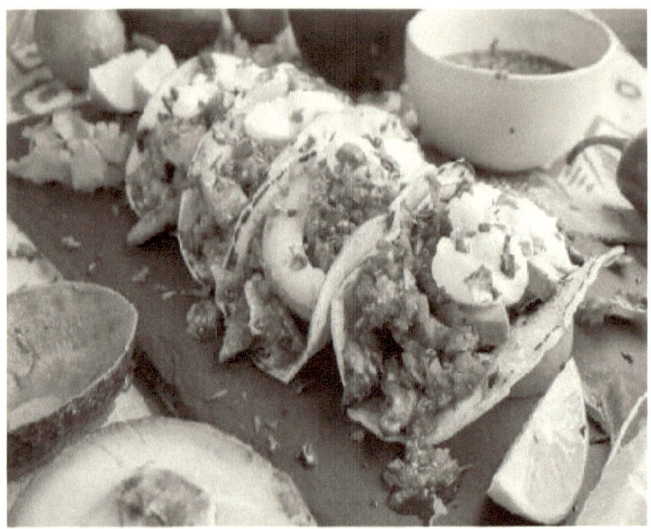

Ingredients :

- 1 pound chicken, cut into bite sized pieces
- 1 tablespoon taco seasoning
- 1 tablespoon oil
- 12 small corn tortillas, warmed
- 1/2 cup salsa verde
- 1 avocado, sliced
- 1/2 cup sour cream (optional)
- 1 tablespoon cilantro, chopped (optional)

Instructions:

1. Marinate the chicken in the mixture of the oil and taco seasoning for 20 minutes to overnight.

2. Cook the chicken in a skillet over medium-high heat until cooked through and lightly golden brown on all sides.

3. Assemble the tacos, and enjoy!

4. Option: Use leftover skillet chicken verde, taco lime grilled chicken, tequila lime grilled chicken, cilantro lime grilled chicken instead of the taco seasoned chicken.

5. Option: Top with your favourite taco toppings!

6. Option: Make the taco seasoned chicken the day before and reheat before adding to the tacos.

Notes : This recipe uses regular corn tortillas, but that's an easy fix. Swap it out for some low-carb tortillas and you'll be on track to a delicious dinner. The salsa on this dish makes it taste so fresh

- **Low-Carb Tikka Masala**

Ingredients :

- 1 yellow onion, peeled and chopped
- 1 Tablespoon butter
- 2 chicken breasts (about 1 pound total), cut into 1/2 inch pieces
- sea salt and pepper
- 2 teaspoons coriander
- 2 teaspoons cumin
- 1 1/2 teaspoons paprika
- 1/2 teaspoon cardamon

- 1/2 teaspoon cayenne pepper

- 1/4 teaspoon nutmeg

- 1 Tablespoon fresh ginger, minced

- 1/4 cup tomato paste

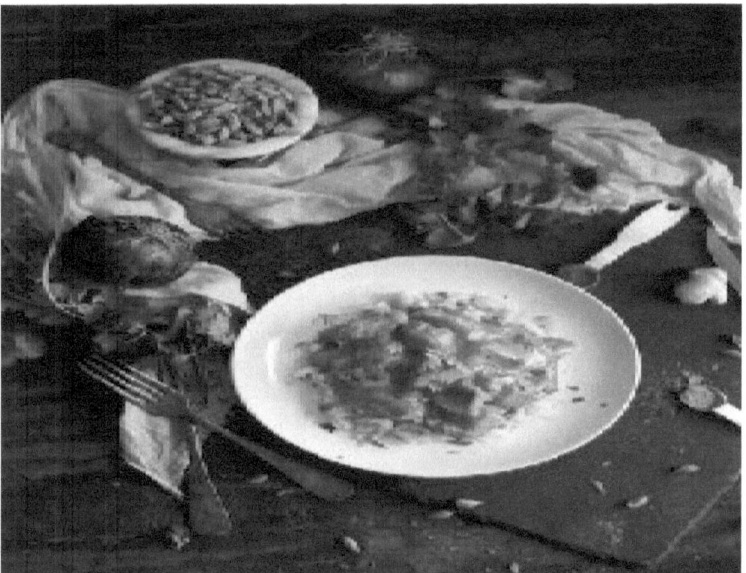

- 1 cup cream

- 1 teaspoon salt

- 1/2 teaspoon freshly ground pepper

- 1/2 cup fresh cilantro finely chopped

Instructions :

1. Heat a large skillet over medium heat. Add butter.

2. When butter stops foaming, add onions to the skillet.

3. Cook onions until they just start browning on the edges. Add chicken and sprinkle with salt and pepper.

4. Brown the chicken pieces on all sides and continue cooking over medium-low heat until they are cooked throughout.

5. Stir in coriander, cumin, paprika, cardamon, cayenne pepper and nutmeg. Cook for about two minutes, stirring constantly, to toast spices.

6. Add fresh ginger, tomato paste and cream to the skillet, stirring to mix thoroughly. Increase heat to medium to bring the mixture to a simmer, then turn the heat to low and continue cooking, stirring occasionally, until sauce thickens to desired consistency.

7. Season with salt and pepper. Stir in cilantro. Taste and adjust seasoning if necessary.

- **Chicken Bacon Ranch Casserole**

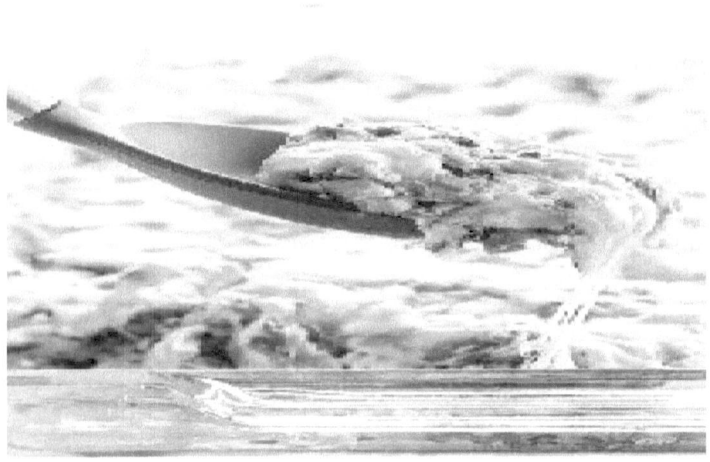

Ingredients :

- Main Ingredients for Chicken Bacon Ranch Casserole
- 2 lb Chicken breast (cooked, cubed or shredded)
- 8 slices Bacon (cooked, chopped)
- 3 cloves Garlic (minced)
- 3/4 cup Ranch dressing
- 1 cup Mozzarella cheese (shredded, divided)
- 1 cup Cheddar cheese (shredded, divided)
- Version 1 with Spinach
- 1 lb Frozen spinach (thawed, squeezed to drain well)

Version 2 with Broccoli

- 4 cup Broccoli (cut into florets)

Instructions :

1. Preheat the oven to 375 degrees F (191 degrees C).

2. If using frozen spinach, thaw and squeeze to drain first. If using broccoli, place it into a pot of water and bring to a boil. Simmer for 1-2 minutes until bright green.

3. Combine the chicken, bacon, drained spinach or broccoli, garlic, ranch dressing, and half of the shredded cheeses in a large bowl. Stir until well incorporated. Transfer to a 9x13 in (23x33 cm) glass or stoneware casserole dish. (Alternatively, you can mix everything directly in the casserole dish.)

4. Top with remaining shredded mozzarella and cheddar cheeses.

5. Bake for about 15 minutes, until hot and bubbly.

- **One Skillet Keto Portuguese Style Chicken**

Ingredients:

- 2 lbs chicken thighs, bone in & skin on
- 1 tbsp avocado oil or olive oil
- 4 slices of a lemon
- 1 ½ cup diced zucchini
- ⅓ cup diced red bell pepper

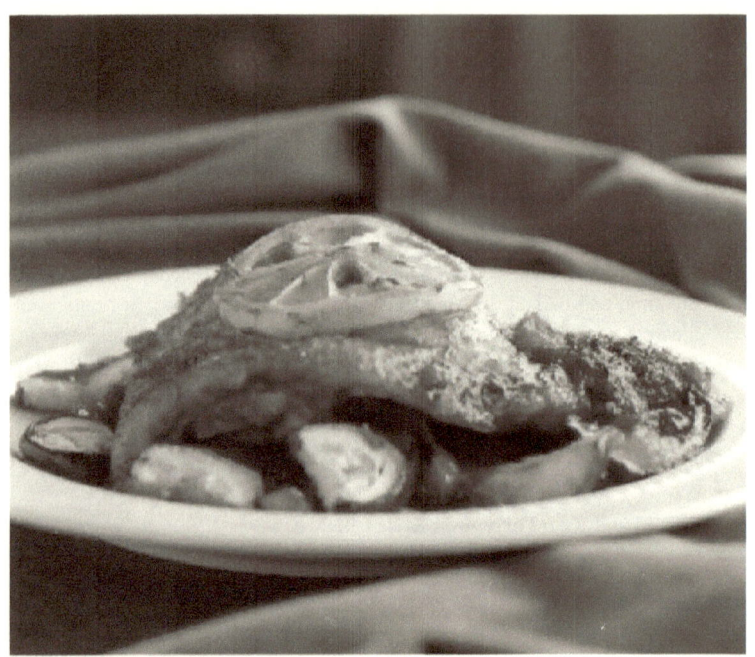

<u>Marinade:</u>

- ¼ cup olive oil
- 3 tbsp lime juice
- 1 tablespoon red wine vinegar
- 3 cloves garlic, peeled and minced
- ¼ tsp crushed red pepper flakes
- 2 tsp paprika
- 1 tsp dried thyme

- ½ tsp salt
- ¼ tsp black pepper
- ¼ tsp black pepper

Instructions :

1. Place all marinade ingredients in a large bowl and whisk until blended. Add chicken thighs to the marinade and turn to coat. Cover the bowl with plastic wrap and refrigerate for 2 to 4 hours.

2. Preheat oven to 400° F(204° C).

3. Heat 1 tbsp avocado oil in a cast iron grill skillet or an oven-safe skillet over medium-high heat.

4. Add chicken to the skillet and brown both sides of chicken until golden brown (about 4 minutes on each side). Once browned, turn off heat.

5. Add zucchini, and red peppers to the skillet arranged around the chicken. Pour any extra marinade from the bowl over chicken and top chicken with lemon slices.

6. Place skillet in the oven and bake for 30 to 35 minutes or until internal temperature of chicken reaches 165 F to 170F.

7. Remove skillet from oven and let rest for 8 minutes and serve.

Keto Dinner Recipes

- **Taco Stuffed Avocados**

Taco Stuffed Avocados. The perfect low carb taco! These avocados are loaded up with the BEST taco meat, cheese, tomatoes, lettuce and a dollop of sour cream. Perfect for an easy lunch or light dinner.

Servings: 6

Ingredients :

- 1 pound ground beef
- 1 tablespoon Chili Powder
- ½ teaspoon Salt
- ¾ teaspoon Cumin
- ½ teaspoon Dried Oregano
- ¼ teaspoon Garlic Powder
- ¼ teaspoon Onion Powder

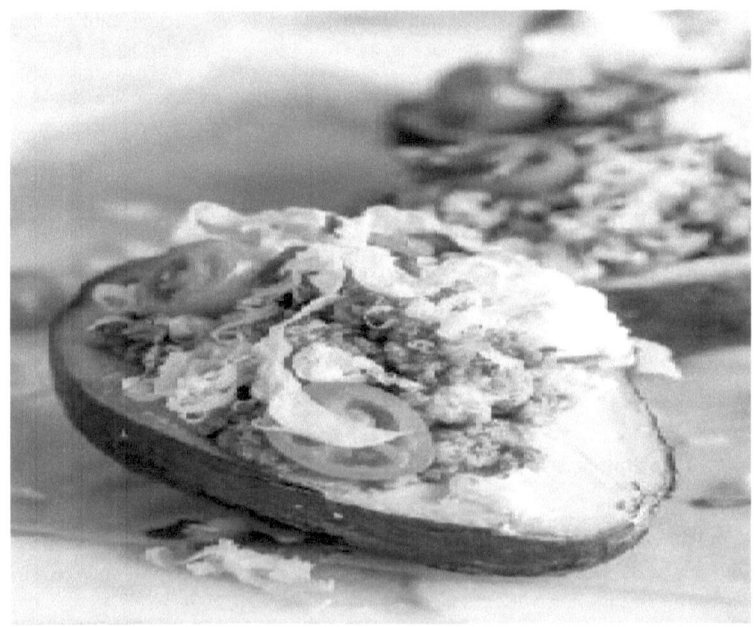

- 4 ounces tomato sauce
- 3 avocados halved
- 1 cup shredded cheddar cheese
- ¼ cup cherry tomatoes sliced
- ¼ cup lettuce shredded

Additional toppings:

- cilantro
- sour cream

Instructions :

1. Add the ground beef to a medium size sauce pan. Cook over medium heat until browned.
2. Drain the grease and add the seasonings and the tomato sauce. Stir to combine. Cook for about 3-4 minutes.
3. Remove the pit from the halved avocados. Load the crater left from the pit with the taco meat. Top with cheese, tomatoes, lettuce, cilantro and sour cream.
4. If you want to make a larger area in the avocado for the toppings, spoon out some of the avocado and set aside to make guacamole! Then fill with toppings.

Notes : Serve with some Cilantro Lime Cauliflower Rice!

- **Spicy Shrimp and Broccoli Mash**

Ingredients:

- 1 tablespoon olive oil
- 1 head broccoli, cut into small florets (about 6 cups)

- 3 cloves garlic, minced
- 3 cups vegetable or chicken broth
- 1 tablespoon heavy cream
- ½ cup parmesan cheese
- 1 teaspoon salt
- 1 tablespoon olive oil
- 1 lb. (450g) raw shrimp, peeled and deveined
- 1 tablespoon minced garlic, or dried garlic

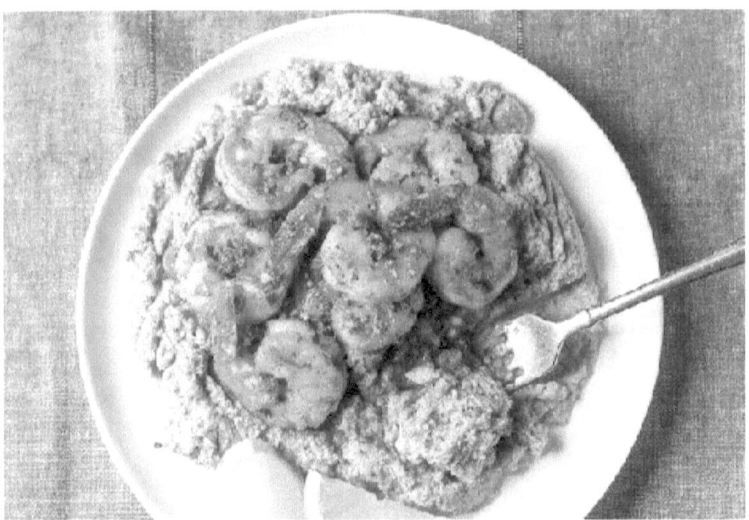

- 1 teaspoon crushed chili pepper flakes
- 1 knob fresh ginger, grated (optional)
- Salt and fresh cracked black pepper

- Lemon wedges, for garnish

Instructions:

1. For the broccoli: Heat the olive oil in a large soup pot. Add the broccoli and garlic. Saute for a minute or two, until the garlic is really fragrant. Add 2 cups broth and simmer for 7 to 10 minutes, until soft.

2. Drain broccoli florets and garlic and transfer to a food processor. Add a tablespoon heavy cream and pulse until smooth. Adjust the consistency by adding few tablespoons of broth if needed. Stir in the salt and parmesan cheese, pulse once more and set aside.

3. For the shrimp: In a large skillet, add the olive oil over medium heat. Make sure to pat the shrimp dry. Add shrimp to the skillet and sprinkle with garlic, salt, pepper, ginger, chili pepper flakes, to taste. Cook for a few minutes on both sides, then add 2 tablespoons water or broth to the pan to deglaze the browned bits and spices to coat the shrimp.

4. Serve the shrimp over a couple spoonfuls of broccoli mash and garnish with lemon wedges. Enjoy!

- **Keto Beef And Broccoli Stir Fry**

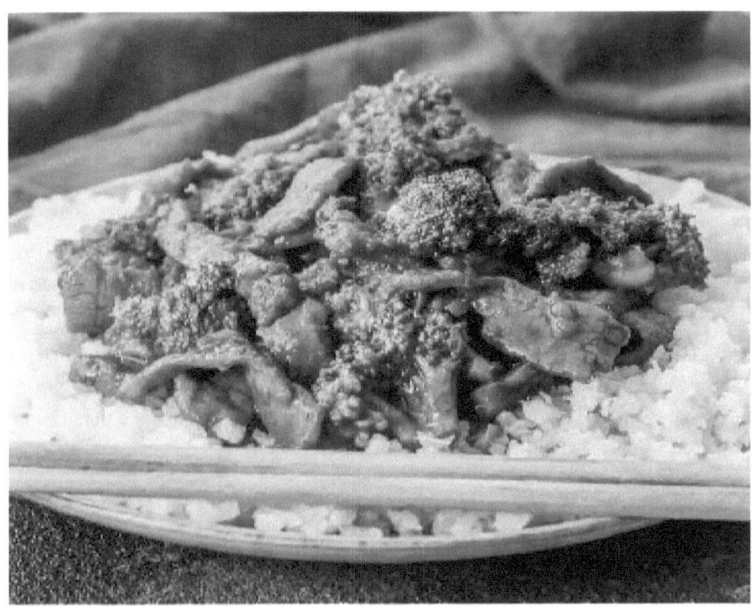

Serving : 2

Ingredients :

- 3/4 pound flank steak sliced into 1/4 inch thick strips
- 4 cups small broccoli florets (about 7 ounces)
- 1/2 cup beef stock
- 1 tablespoon corn starch
- 1 tablespoon canola oil
- For the sauce:
- 1/3 cup low-sodium soy sauce
- 3-5 tablespoons sweetener (see post for options)

Instructions :

1. Toss the sliced beef in a large bowl with corn starch until well-coated. Set aside.

2. Heat canola oil in a pan over medium heat for a few minutes or until hot.

3. Add sliced beef and cook until it browns, less than 5 minutes, stirring frequently. Transfer to a plate and set aside.

4. Add broccoli florets to the pan and stir. Add beef broth. Let simmer until the broccoli is tender, about 10 minutes, stirring occasionally.

5. While waiting for the broccoli to cook, combine all sauce ingredients in a sauce pan. Stir the ingredients together over medium-low heat until it starts to simmer, about 5 minutes. Keep the sauce warm over low heat as you wait for the broccoli to cook.

6. Return beef to the pan and pour the sauce on top. Stir until everything is coated with the sauce. Bring to a simmer and cook for another few minutes.

7. Season with salt and pepper to taste, if needed.

8. Serve immediately, optionally pairing with cooked cauliflower rice. Drizzle sauce on top.

- **Sheet-Pan Salsa Chicken with Spaghetti Squash**

This well-balanced keto meal combines the flavors of red salsa chicken with delicious squash noodles, for an out-of-this-world keto dinner recipe.

Ingredients:

- 1 spaghetti squash
- 3 skinless, boneless chicken breasts, split in 2
- 1 can peeled tomatoes

- 1 onion, finely minced
- 5 garlic cloves, finely minced
- 1 Jalapeno, diced

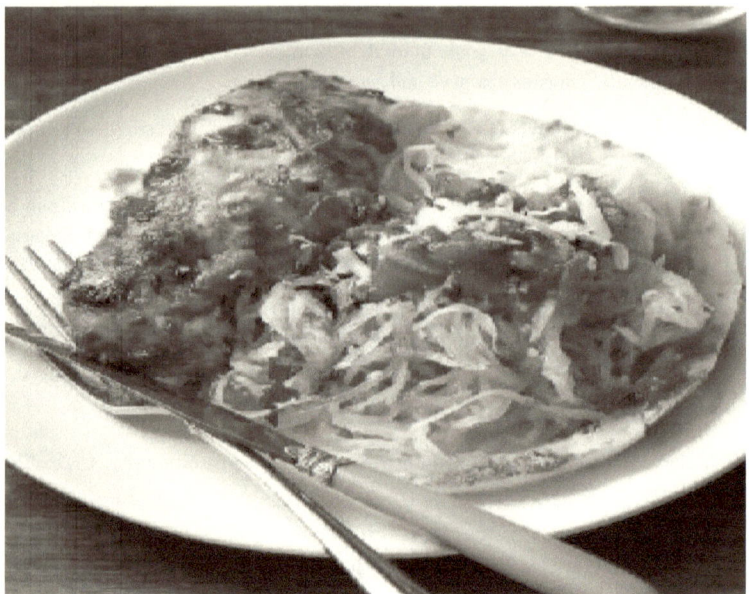

- 1 handful cilantro, chopped
- 1 bouillon cube, crumbled
- 1 coffee spoon ground cumin
- 1 teaspoon Italian seasoning
- 1 handful Italian four cheese mix

Instructions:

1. Preheat your oven to 450°F (230°C) and line a baking sheet with parchment paper. Rinse and cut the spaghetti squash in half, remove seed, then cut into 1/2 inch rings. Arrange the rings on the baking sheet, sprinkle with salt and pepper.

2. In a bowl, combine tomatoes, diced jalapeño, garlic, onion, cilantro, crumbled bouillon cube, Italian seasoning, cumin and set aside.

3. Season chicken breasts with salt and pepper and arrange on top of the spaghetti squash rings. Drizzle generously with the tomato salsa and sprinkle with cheese.

4. Bake in the preheated oven for 15-20 minutes, until golden and cooked through. You can finish with 5 minutes in grill/broiler mode. Serve hot, directly from the pan after sprinkling with additional cheese and cilantro.

- **Easy Eggless Salmon Patties**

Salmon patties are great to have on the ketogenic diet, but sometimes they taste too eggy.

Fortunately, this recipe is revolutionary in that you don't need eggs at all.

Serving : 6 Patties

Ingredients :

- 6 tablespoons water
- 2 tablespoons golden flaxseed meal
- 18 oz Wild Pink Salmon (about 3 cans), well drained (see notes)
- ½ cup almond meal
- 1/2 cup fresh parsley ,chopped
- 1 shallot ,finely chopped

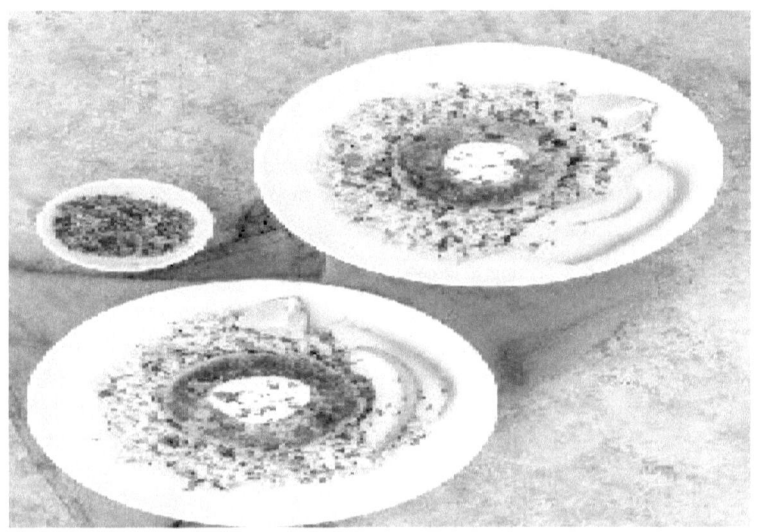

- 1 green onion ,sliced
- 1 teaspoon salt
- 1 teaspoon garlic powder
- ½ teaspoon dill
- ¼ teaspoon black pepper
- 2 tablespoons lime juice
- 2 tablespoons olive oil

Instructions :

1. Add flaxseed meal and water to a small bowl and stir. Let rest for 5 minutes to thicken.

2. Flake the salmon apart in a medium bowl. Add almond meal, parsley, shallot, green onion, salt, garlic powder, dill, black pepper, lime juice, and the flaxseed mixture. Mix until well incorporated.

3. Form into 6 patties. I use a ½ cup measuring cup to portion the mixture and to make sure all the patties are the same size.

4. Heat olive oil over medium heat in a nonstick skillet. Fry the patties for 4- 5 minutes on each side until golden brown and crispy.

5. Serve with cilantro lime cauliflower rice, if desired

* **Creamy Tuscan Garlic Chicken**

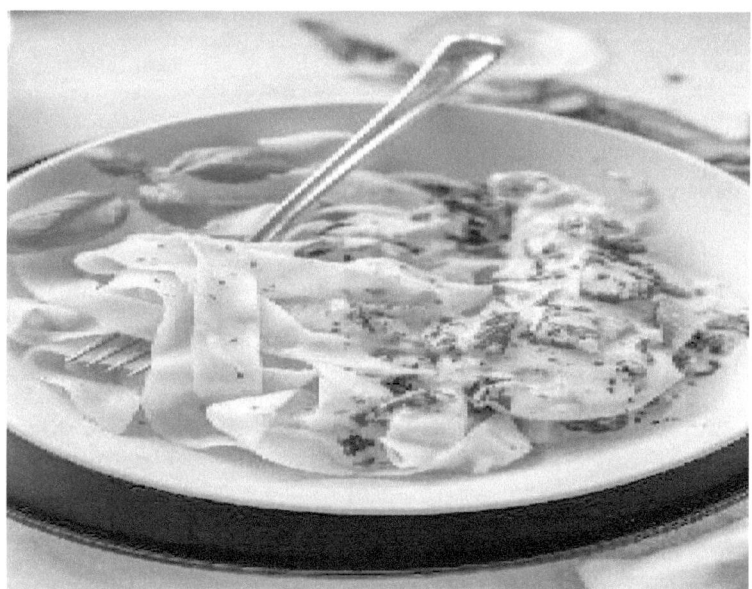

This delicious keto recipe made with chicken, garlic, spinach, and cream tastes like you're in a restaurant.

Ingredients :

- 1-2 tablespoons extra-virgin olive oil
- 1/4 cup all-purpose flour
- 4 boneless skinless chicken breasts thinly-sliced (about 1-1.5 pounds) (see note 1)
- 2-3 teaspoons kosher salt
- a few turns of freshly-ground black pepper
- 4 cloves garlic minced
- 1/2 cup chicken broth
- 3/4 cup heavy cream
- 1 teaspoon Italian seasoning
- 1/2 cup Parmesan cheese grated
- 1-2 cups fresh spinach roughly chopped
- 1/2 cup sun-dried tomatoes roughly chopped
- pasta for serving

Instructions :

1. In a large skillet, warm olive oil over medium-high heat. Place flour in a small bowl or plate. Lightly sprinkle each side of the chicken breasts with kosher salt and black pepper, then dredge each side lightly through the flour. Shake off any excess, then place chicken breasts in the warm pan. Cook for 3-4 minutes on each side, just until browned and no longer pink in the center. Remove chicken to a plate and set aside.

2. If the skillet is dry, add a tiny bit more olive oil, followed by the garlic. Cook for about 1 minute, just until fragrant. Add chicken broth, and scrape any browned bits from the bottom of the skillet.

3. Add cream, Italian seasoning, and Parmesan cheese. Cook over medium heat for 5-7 minutes, stirring frequently, until the sauce visibly thickens.

4. Stir in spinach and sun-dried tomatoes, and simmer for 1-2 minutes, until spinach wilts.

5. Add chicken back to the skillet, spoon a bit of sauce over each piece, and serve with pasta or other sides as desired.

TIPS

1. If possible, take your chicken breasts out of the fridge and let them rest at room temperature for 10-15 minutes before you start cooking. This helps them to cook more evenly, so the inside is done just as the outside gets nice and browned.

2. In a pinch, you could sub 1 teaspoon garlic powder for the freshly minced cloves.

3. If using oil-packed sun-dried tomatoes, drain and try to pat a little bit of the oil off of them before chopping and mixing in with the sauce.

4. This is a rich and very flavorful sauce, so even if serving with pasta, we find a little goes a long way, and don't typically coat all of the pasta in sauce as you might want to with, say, a lighter marinara or the like.

- **One Pan Keto Sausage Dinner**

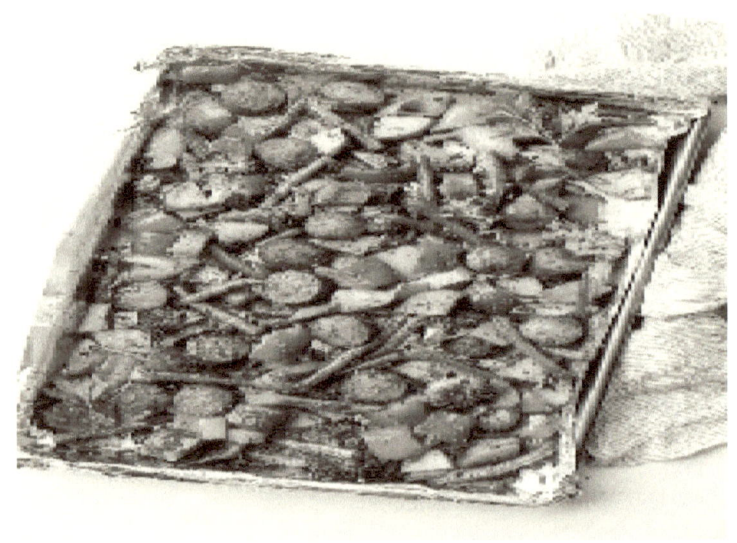

Ingredients :

- 2 cups (~1 small) red potato
- 3/4ths pound green beans
- 1 large head of broccoli (~ 1 and 1/2 cups)
- 1 and 1/2 cups chopped bell peppers 2 large or 6-7 mini sweet bell peppers
- 9 ounces smoked sausage I use turkey or chicken, not ground sausage
- 6 tablespoons olive oil
- 1/4 teaspoon red pepper flakes optional
- 1 teaspoon paprika
- 1/2 teaspoon garlic powder
- 1 tablespoon dried oregano

- 1 tablespoon dried parsley
- 1/4 teaspoon salt
- 1/4 teaspoon pepper

Instructions:

1. Preheat the oven to 400 degrees F.
2. Line a large sheet pan with foil or parchment paper.
3. Prep the veggies: chop the red potatoes (pretty small pieces here so they will be tender in time), trim the green beans and halve, chop the broccoli, chop the peppers into thick squares, and coin the sausage in thick slices.
4. Place all the veggies and sausage on a sheet pan. Pour the olive oil and all the spices on top. Toss to evenly coat all the veggies and meat.
5. Bake 15 minutes, remove from the oven and flip/stir all the veggies around. Return to the oven and bake for another 10-15 minutes or until vegetables are crisp tender and sausage is browned.
6. If desired, sprinkle freshly grated Parmesan cheese over the veggies and sausage as soon as they come out of the oven.
7. Enjoy with rice or *q*uinoa and fresh parsley if desired.

Serve with: fresh parsley, quinoa/rice, lots of freshly grated Parmesan cheese

- **Spiced Crispy Chicken Skin Tostad**

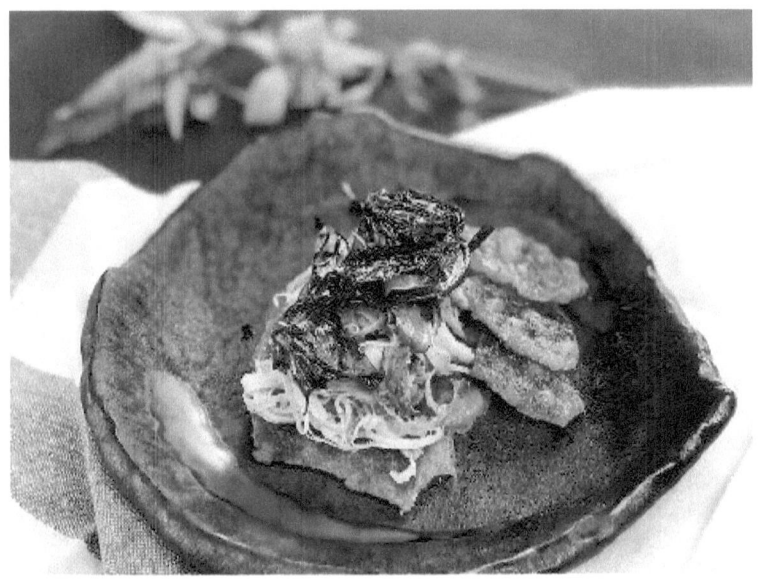

Ingredients :

- 1 ½ teaspoons five spice powder

- ¼ teaspoon chili powder

- 4 medium chicken quarters

- 3 medium cloves garlic, grated

- 2 teaspoons grated ginger

- 1 tablespoon tamari

- 1 tablespoon Shaoxing wine

- 2 teaspoons erythritol

- 2 tablespoons olive oil

- 1 cup fresh basil leaves

- Salt and Pepper, to taste

Directions :

- Pre-heat oven to 350 degrees. In a small bowl, combine salt and pepper, half of the five-spice powder, and chili powder. Mix well and set aside; this will be your spice salt.

- Carefully pull chicken skin off thigh over leg bone. The easiest way to do this is to maneuver your thumb in between the chicken skin and meat.

- Snip the chicken skin with scissors. Trim the chicken skin using knife or cutters into bite-sized portions. [The chicken skin will shrink, so make allowances.]

- Season generously with the spice salt.

- Layer a baking sheet tray with parchment paper, chicken skin, and then an additional layer of parchment paper.

- Place an additional baking sheet on top of the final layer of parchment paper. This ensures that the chicken skin will not stick or curl while baking.

- Bake the chicken skin for 30-35 minutes. Remove chicken skin from the oven and set aside to cool.

- In the Instant Pot, add skinned chicken quarters with garlic, ginger, tamari, Shaoxing, sweetener, salt, and remaining five spice. Set the Instant Pot to manual high for 30 minutes. Perform a manual release when it's done, then turn off the Instant Pot and let the chicken cool just long enough to handle.

- Shred chicken and set aside.

- Pre-heat a pan on the stove. then add olive oil to it. Once the olive oil is hot, scatter basil leaves and cook until translucent.

- Remove the basil leaves and drain on paper towel. Set aside. Using the same pan, add shredded chicken.

- Cook the chicken to give it some color and bring it back up to temp.

- To serve, top spiced crispy chicken skin with shredded chicken, remaining spiced salt, and basil.

- **Keto Instant Pot Crack Chicken Recipe**

Rich, creamy, and full of flavor, this Keto Instant Pot Crack Chicken Recipe is sure to be a favorite family dinner.

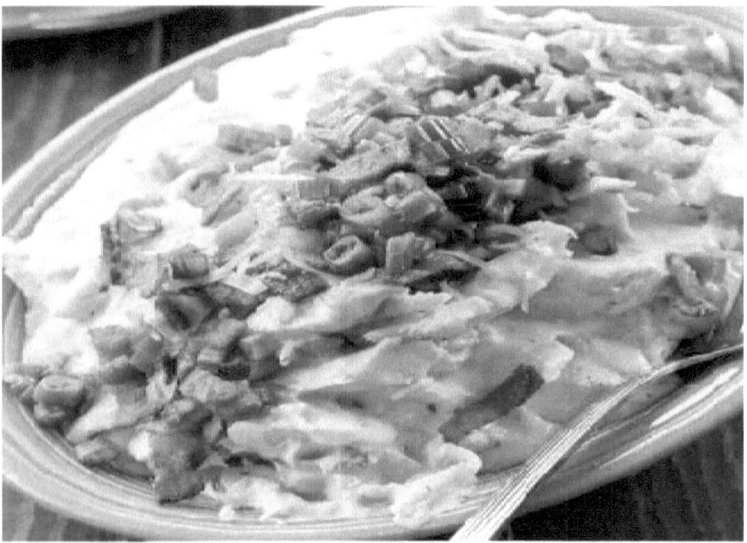

Ingredients :

- 2 slices bacon, chopped

- 2 lbs (910 g) boneless, skinless chicken breasts
- 2 (8 oz/227 g) blocks cream cheese
- ½ cup (120 ml) water
- 2 tablespoons apple cider vinegar
- 1 tablespoon dried chives
- 1½ teaspoons garlic powder
- 1½ teaspoons onion powder
- 1 teaspoon crushed red pepper flakes
- 1 teaspoon dried dill
- ¼ teaspoon salt
- ¼ teaspoon black pepper
- ½ cup (2 oz/57 g) shredded cheddar
- 1 scallion, green and white parts, thinly sliced

Directions :

- Turn pressure cooker on, press 'Saute', and wait 2 minutes for the pot to heat up. Add the chopped bacon and cook until crispy. Transfer to a plate and set aside. Press "Cancel" to stop sautéing. (See Note.)
- Add the chicken, cream cheese, water, vinegar, chives, garlic powder, onion powder, crushed red pepper flakes, dill, salt, and black pepper to the pot. Turn the pot on Manual, High Pressure for 15 minutes and then do a quick release.
- Use tongs to transfer the chicken to a large plate, shred it with 2 forks, and return it back to the pot.
- Stir in the cheddar cheese.

- Top with the crispy bacon and scallion, and serve.

• **Instant pot lemon chicken with garlic**

This Instant Pot Lemon Chicken with Garlic is an easy low carb / keto-friendly meal for spring. Best of all, this pressure cooker chicken recipe cooks up tender, juicy and full of flavor!

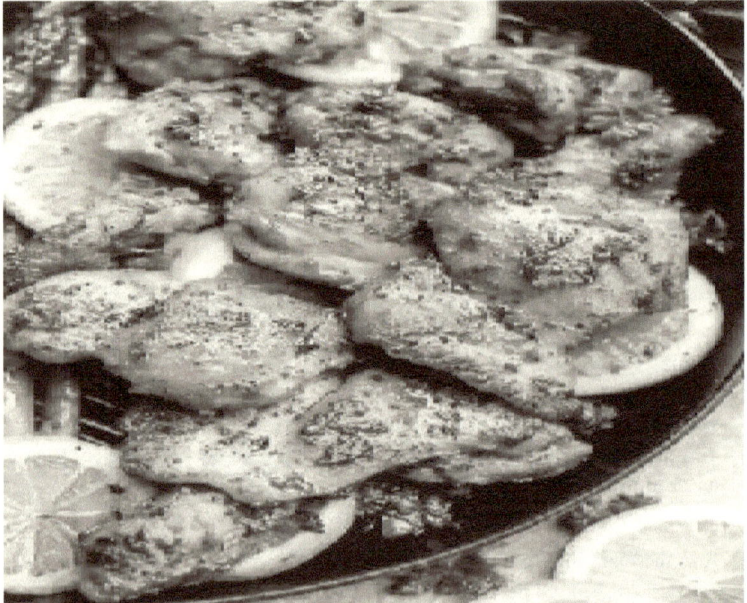

Ingredients :

- 8 tablespoons butter

- ½ cup coconut flour
- 4 cups chicken broth
- 4 teaspoons chili powder
- 1 tablespoon ground cumin
- 1 tablespoons garlic powder
- 1 teaspoon salt
- Pepper to taste
- 2.5 pounds boneless, skinless, chicken breasts
- 1 (10-ounce) can diced tomatoes with green chilies
- 1 medium jalapeno, diced with seeds removed
- ½ cup heavy whipping cream
- 1 ½ teaspoons xanthan gum
- 2 cups shredded Mexican blend cheese
- Chopped cilantro, to taste

Directions :

- Turn the Instant Pot on to the low saute setting. Melt the butter.
- Whisk in the coconut flour and cook for a few minutes.
- Stir in the chicken broth. Add chili powder, ground cumin, garlic powder, salt, and pepper.
- Place the chicken breasts into the slow cooker.
- Add the green chilies and jalapeno.

- Seal the Instant Pot then pressure cook for 15 minutes. Once it's done do a manual release.
- Stir in the heavy whipping cream and xanthan gum, then mix in the cheese. You can use tongs to break the chicken up into smaller pieces, or remove and slice then add back to the pot.
- Serve with chopped cilantro and additional cheese if desired.

- **Crab Stuffed Mushrooms with cream cheese**

An easy recipe for crab stuffed mushrooms with cream cheese. Low carb, keto, and gluten free.

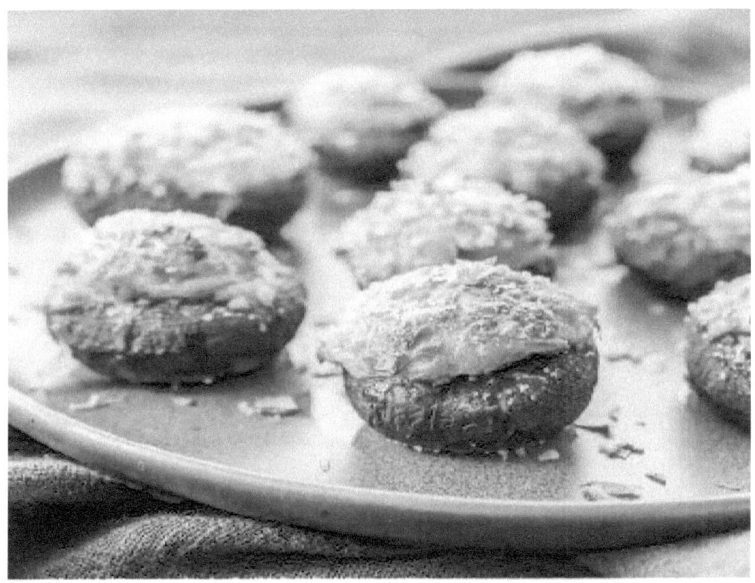

Ingredients :

- 20 ounces cremini (baby bella) mushrooms (20-25 individual mushrooms)
- 2 tablespoons finely grated parmesan cheese
- 1 tablespoon chopped fresh parsley
- salt

Filling:

- 4 ounces cream cheese softened to room temperature

- 4 ounces crab meat finely chopped
- 5 cloves garlic minced
- 1 teaspoon dried oregano
- 1/2 teaspoon paprika
- 1/2 teaspoon black pepper
- 1/4 teaspoon salt

Directions :

- Preheat the oven to 400 F. Prepare a baking sheet lined with parchment paper.
- Snap stems from mushrooms, discarding the stems and placing the mushroom caps on the baking sheet 1 inch apart from each other. Season the mushroom caps with salt.
- In a large mixing bowl, combine all filling ingredients and stir until well-mixed without any lumps of cream cheese. Stuff the mushroom caps with the mixture. Evenly sprinkle parmesan cheese on top of the stuffed mushrooms.
- Bake at 400 F until the mushrooms are very tender and the stuffing is nicely browned on top, about 30 minutes. Top with parsley and serve while hot.

Conclusion

Thank you so much for securing a copy of my cookbook. I hope you have gotten adequate information towards creating your favorite keto recipes for weight loss .

Stay healthy!!!!

©2019 By: Damon Axe

www.ingramcontent.com/pod-product-compliance
Lightning Source LLC
Chambersburg PA
CBHW020317290526
45785CB00007B/2824

* 9 7 8 1 0 7 0 6 2 8 6 4 6 *